CLINICAL GUIDE TO ALCOHOL TREATMENT

The Community Reinforcement Approach

THE GUILFORD SUBSTANCE ABUSE SERIES
Howard T. Blane and Thomas R. Kosten, *Editors*

Recent Volumes

Clinical Guide to Alcohol Treatment: The Community Reinforcement Approach
ROBERT J. MEYERS and JANE ELLEN SMITH

Psychotherapy and Substance Abuse: A Practitioner's Handbook
ARNOLD M. WASHTON, *Editor*

Introduction to Addictive Behaviors. DENNIS L. THOMBS

Treating Alcohol Problems: Marital and Family Interventions
TIMOTHY J. O'FARRELL, *Editor*

Clinical Work with Substance-Abusing Clients
SHULAMITH LALA ASHENBERG STRAUSSNER, *Editor*

Clean Start: An Outpatient Program for Initiating Cocaine Recovery
WILLIAM E. McAULIFFE and JEFFREY ALBERT

Clinician's Guide to Cocaine Addiction: Theory, Research and Treatment
THOMAS R. KOSTEN and HERBERT D. KLEBER, *Editors*

Alcohol Tolerance and Social Drinking: Learning the Consequences
MURIEL VOGEL-SPROTT

Removing the Roadblocks: Group Psychotherapy
with Substance Abusers and Family Members
MARSHA VANNICELLI

Group Psychotherapy with Adult Children of Alcoholics:
Treatment Techniques and Countertransference Considerations
MARSHA VANNICELLI

Children of Alcoholics: Critical Perspectives
MICHAEL WINDLE and JOHN S. SEARLES, *Editors*

Preventing AIDS in Drug Users and Their Sexual Partners
JAMES L. SORENSEN, LAURIE A. WERMUTH, DAVID R. GIBSON,
KYUNG-HEE CHOI, JOSEPH R. GUYDISH, and STEVEN L. BATKI

Alcohol in Human Violence; KAI PERNANEN

Clinical Textbook of Addictive Disorders
RICHARD J. FRANCES and SHELDON I. MILLER, *Editors*

Drinking and Driving: Advances in Research and Prevention
R. JEAN WILSON and ROBERT E. MANN, *Editors*

Addiction and the Vulnerable Self:
Modified Dynamic Group Therapy for Substance Abusers
EDWARD J. KHANTZIAN, KURT S. HALLIDAY, and WILLIAM E.
McAULIFFE

Alcohol and the Family: Research and Clinical Perspectives
R. LORRAINE COLLINS, KENNETH E. LEONARD, and JOHN S. SEARLES,
Editors

CLINICAL GUIDE
TO
ALCOHOL TREATMENT

The Community Reinforcement Approach

ROBERT J. MEYERS

JANE ELLEN SMITH

THE GUILFORD PRESS
New York   London

© 1995 The Guilford Press
A Division of Guilford Publications, Inc.
72 Spring Street, New York, NY 10012

Printed in the United States of America

This book is printed on acid-free paper.

Last digit is print number: 9 8 7 6 5 4 3

Library of Congress Cataloging-in-Publication Data

Meyers, Robert J.
    Clinical guide to alcohol treatment : the community reinforcement
approach / by Robert J. Meyers, Jane Ellen Smith.
        p.   cm. — (The guilford substance abuse series)
    Includes bibliographical references and index.
    ISBN 0-89862-857-1
1. Alcoholism—Treatment.   2. Behavior therapy.   3. Alcoholics-
-Counseling of.   4. Social networks—Therapeutic use.   5. Operant
conditioning.   I. Smith, Jane Ellen.   II. Title.   III. Series
        [DNLM: 1. Alcoholism—therapy.   2. Behavior Therapy—methods.
    3. Counseling.   4. Reinforcement (Psychology).   WM 274 M613c 1995]
    RC565, M427   1995
    616.88'106—dc20
DNLM/DLC
for Library of Congress   95-546
                                                                              CIP

To all my friends and colleagues from the early days in Southern Illinois— Nate A., Floyd C., Bobby S., Kevin F., Wendy B., Paul S., Jackie B., Connie B., Fran C., Dave M., Jo N., and Mark Godley—who remained patient and supportive throughout those exciting but difficult times. And a special thanks to John Mallams for his mentorship early in my career and for his help on this project.

RJM

To the dedicated faculty in the Psychology Department at the State University of New York at Binghamton . . . for teaching me the value of the scientist–practitioner model.

JES

Foreword_____

When I first met Bob Meyers a decade ago, I knew relatively little about the community reinforcement approach (CRA), but it was clear to me from the research of Azrin's group in the 1970s that the CRA was a promising strategy for treating alcohol problems. Unlike many approaches, it also seemed to be most effective with what would be regarded as "poor prognosis" groups—more severely dependent and less socially stable individuals. Yet, in spite of this rather strong track record in outcome research, the CRA languished, almost completely unused and unknown.

Perhaps the largest obstacle to implementation of the CRA was the lack of a clear set of therapeutic guidelines for its application. The original research reports included only a brief sketch of how one actually does CRA treatment, and the Illinois team that had given birth to this approach had scattered to new tasks and locations. Bob's arrival as a staff member at the Center on Alcoholism, Substance Abuse, and Addictions (CASAA) at the University of New Mexico gave rise to a clinical research program focusing on the CRA as a treatment strategy for alcohol and other drug problems. Over the years in clinical trials at CASAA, treatment procedures and manuals began to take shape, building on the pioneering work of the original Azrin group of which Bob had been a part. Under his direction, the clinical team at CASAA developed a clearer understanding of CRA philosophy, procedures, and practicalities.

No longer is the CRA an unknown method. Several research teams are now actively studying this clinical approach. Training and research on CRA have spread not only through the United States, but as far as New Zealand, Poland, and the Netherlands. Major grant funding for CRA studies has been provided by the National Institute on Alcohol Abuse and Alcoholism, and the National Institute on Drug Abuse. It was included in *Broadening the Base of Treatment for Alcohol Problems*, a 1990 major report from the Institute of Medicine of the National Academy of Sciences. Many of the procedures included in the original CRA—motivational preparation, behavioral marital therapy, communication skills training, and stress management—have subsequently been shown separately in clinical trials to be important and effective elements in treatment. Yet the CRA itself remains an approach unfamiliar to many clinicians in the field.

I hope this book will change all that. It is the first complete and authoritative statement on clinical practice of the community reinforcement approach. The collaboration of Bob Meyers with Dr. Jane Ellen Smith, our Director of Clinical Training at the University of New Mexico, has produced a clear, engaging, and accurate description of the hows and whys of this exciting approach. The outcome data to date are solid indeed. The real gift of this volume, however, is that it makes the CRA understandable, accessible, and practicable for clinicians.

Many have decried the large gap between research and practice in the field of alcohol/drug abuse. The fact is that most of the treatments used in practice have a relatively poor track record in outcome research, whereas well-substantiated methods like the CRA remain largely unused. The responsibility for this gap lies as much with researchers as with clinicians. Reports of favorable treatment outcomes often lack sufficient information to allow clinicians to use new treatment methods in practice. Such was certainly the case with the CRA. This book is the kind of work that builds bridges, and allows the findings of years of careful clinical research to finally receive everyday application. It is a pleasing marriage of research and treatment, science and practice. Such collaborations are vital for improving health care in the area of alcohol/drug problems, because the perspectives of clinicians can improve the quality of treatment research, and it is sound research that ultimately points us toward the best clinical strategies for alleviating human suffering.

WILLIAM R. MILLER, PH.D.
Professor of Psychology and Psychiatry
Director, Research Division, CASAA
The University of New Mexico
Albuquerque, New Mexico

Contents

Chapter 1

History of the Community Reinforcement Approach
1

Chapter 2
CRA Assessment
17

Chapter 3
Sobriety Sampling
42

Chapter 4
Disulfiram Use Within CRA
57

Chapter 5
CRA Treatment Plan
80

ix

Chapter 6
Behavioral Skills Training
102

Chapter 7
Additional CRA Techniques
121

Chapter 8
Social and Recreational Counseling
138

Chapter 9
CRA Marital Therapy
147

Chapter 10
CRA Relapse Prevention
180

Chapter 11
The Big Picture
196

References
204

Index
207

CLINICAL GUIDE TO ALCOHOL TREATMENT

The Community Reinforcement Approach

1

History of the Community Reinforcement Approach

The Community Reinforcement Approach (CRA) is a broad spectrum behavioral treatment approach for substance abuse problems. It was developed to utilize social, recreational, familial, and vocational reinforcers to aid clients in the recovery process. CRA acknowledges the powerful role of environmental contingencies in encouraging or discouraging drinking, and thus attempts to rearrange these contingencies such that sober behavior is more rewarding than drinking behavior. CRA blends this operant model with a social systems approach. The overall philosophy is to use the community to reward nondrinking behavior so that the client makes healthy lifestyle changes.

The Earliest CRA Trials

Azrin and his colleagues demonstrated in three well-designed alcohol studies that CRA was superior to standard treatment procedures. In the original matched-control study (Hunt & Azrin, 1973), 8 alcoholic inpatients were selected and then matched individually with 8 others on age, education, drinking history, family stability, and employment record. Random assignment determined which member of each pair was to receive CRA counseling. Subjects in the Standard Treatment group received the hospital's traditional Alcoholics Anonymous (AA) program. Based on the early Jellinek disease model of alcoholism (E. M. Jellinek, 1960), it revolved around the 12 steps of AA. The 25 one-hour instructional sessions covered such topics as (1) basic AA procedures, (2) the problems of alcoholics, (3) typical alcoholics' behavior, (4) medical complications of alcoholism, and (5) alcohol-related sexual problems. Most therapists delivering this treatment were recovering alcoholics who fully embraced the AA model.

The subjects assigned to the CRA group received the same standard treatment in addition to the basic CRA procedures. These included (1) job counseling, (2) social and leisure counseling, (3) assistance in accessing nondrinking reinforcers, (4) an alcohol-free social club, and (5) relapse prevention in the form of home visits by the CRA counselors. Married clients also received behavioral marital therapy.

Posttreatment results showed that subjects who received CRA counseling spent significantly less time drinking and in institutions than did Standard Treatment subjects, and significantly more time working and being with their families. More specifically, the 6-month follow-up results demonstrated that CRA group members were drinking 14% of the follow-up days in contrast to the Standard Treatment group's report of 79% of the days. Striking results were noted in the area of unemployment as well, with the CRA subjects being unemployed only 5% of follow-up days, and the Standard Treatment subjects reporting unemployment 62% of the follow-up time. Additionally, the CRA group only spent an average of 16% of follow-up nights away from their families, while the Standard Treatment group participants spent 36% of follow-up nights away. With regard to institutionalization, CRA group members were hospitalized 2% of follow-up days, as contrasted with 27% of follow-up days for the Standard Treatment group. None of the CRA subjects got divorced or separated during the 6-month follow-up period, while 50% of the couples in the Standard Treatment group either divorced or separated during that same time.

Although the results had to be interpreted cautiously due to the limited number of subjects, this experiment was considered extremely important for a variety of reasons. To begin with, it was one of the few alcohol treatment studies of the time that included a control group. Also, the CRA subjects' dramatic improvements were not restricted to their drastically altered drinking patterns, but were evidenced in many other areas of their lives as well. And finally, CRA offered an interesting new conceptualization of alcoholism etiology that relied upon operant reinforcement theory.

A second CRA trial showed similar results (Azrin, 1976). This study was an extension and modification of the first design, as it introduced four new procedures to the already established CRA interventions. These included (1) a prescription for disulfiram, (2) a compliance program that monitored and reinforced subjects for taking the disulfiram, (3) an early warning monitoring program to signal developing difficulties, and (4) a buddy system as a source of continued social support. Further modifications to the original CRA package entailed the delivery of treatment in a group as opposed to an individual format, and the utilization of several different counselors. The control group received the hospital's standard services. These included (1) education about the dangers of alcohol, (2) both individual and group counseling, (3) advice to take disulfiram, and (4) strong encouragement to join AA. The study was conducted with inpatients using a matched-control design. Nine pairs of subjects were matched on five variables: job satisfaction, job stability, family stability, social life, and drinking history. The member of the pair to receive CRA treatment was determined randomly.

The CRA group showed superior outcomes relative to their control counterparts at the 6-month follow-up. Follow-up time spent drinking averaged 2% for the CRA group and 55% for the control group. Unemployment time was reported as 20% for the CRA group and 56% for the control group. The CRA subjects spent nights away from their families an average of 7% of the time, in comparison to 67% for the control group. And finally, the CRA subjects were never institutionalized, while the control group averaged 45% of their time hospitalized. Statistically each of these comparisons was significantly different. Results for the 2-year follow-up were equally impressive, as the abstention rate for all CRA subjects was 90%.

The results of this second study are particularly noteworthy, given that the median counseling time was only 30 hours, as compared to 50 hours in the first study. Furthermore, the results from all three of the CRA counselors were similar, suggesting that the effectiveness was due to CRA procedures, and not to individual differences in counselor style. The study also was remarkable for its introduction of several novel procedures, including a disulfiram compliance program and an early warning system. And while this second study could be criticized as well for its small sample size, this matter was addressed in later designs.

Application of CRA to Outpatients

The third CRA study was the first one to utilize outpatients (Azrin, Sisson, Meyers, & Godley, 1982). Its main purpose was to examine the contribution of the disulfiram compliance program introduced in the last study (Azrin, 1976) by contrasting it with the traditional procedure for dispensing disulfiram. A second purpose was to test a much abbreviated version of CRA by limiting therapy time to about 5 hours.

Eligible subjects were randomly assigned to one of three treatment conditions: Traditional, Disulfiram Assurance, and CRA Plus Disulfiram Assurance. The Traditional group (n = 14) consisted of 12-step counseling plus a disulfiram prescription. Counselors relied upon (1) reviewing the Jellinek chart (E.M. Jellinek, 1960), (2) showing the Father Martin film *Chalk Talk* (Martin, 1972), and (3) discussing the AA philosophy. Therapists also used a behavioral procedure to ensure that all subjects actually attended AA meetings. The second group, Disulfiram Assurance (n = 15), received this same program, but in addition all subjects and their Concerned Others were instructed in a specific disulfiram compliance procedure. Not only did this procedure entail components of monitoring and reinforcement for disulfiram use, but it also involved practice role-plays of how to handle days on which the subject might be opposed to taking disulfiram. The Concerned Other received communication skills training in order to be prepared to respond appropriately in these situations. Since this group was really a combination of the traditional 12-step treatment and those CRA procedures related to disulfiram compliance, it was expected to produce an outcome midway between that of the other two groups.

The third group, the complete CRA package including Disulfiram Assurance (n = 14), utilized the CRA procedures introduced in the earlier studies as well as several new ones. These included: (1) motivational counseling (Sobriety Sampling), (2) disulfiram administration during the first session, (3) drink-refusal training, and (4) relaxation training. CRA subjects received an average of five therapy sessions, in addition to Job Club visits and phone contacts. Home visits were not conducted during this study.

The results were as predicted, with the two groups that included disulfiram assurance components reporting the highest abstinence rates overall. More specifically, although all three groups achieved almost complete abstinence during the first month of treatment, differences emerged throughout the remainder of the 6-month follow-up. The Disulfiram Assurance group evidenced a steady decrease in both disulfiram use and abstinence rates. During the sixth month of the follow-up, the mean abstention rate for the group was 74% of the days. In contrast, the CRA Plus Disulfiram Assurance group reported an average of less than one drinking day per month during each of the 6 months, or an abstention rate of 97% of the days for the last month. A closer look at the data revealed that the couples within the Disulfiram Assurance group performed much better than the single subjects, even to the point of matching the CRA Plus Disulfiram Assurance group's success on several variables. In terms of the Traditional group's outcome, disulfiram usage dropped out entirely after the third month, and abstinence rates declined accordingly. At the time of the final month of the 6-month follow-up, the Traditional group members were abstinent only 45% of the days. And although statistically significant differences were not detected between the three groups' unemployment rates at the 6-month follow-up, clinically noteworthy differences were found when just the Traditional and the CRA Plus Disulfiram Assurance groups were contrasted. The former group reported being unemployed approximately 36% of the month, and the latter only 7%.

This study was remarkable for its demonstrated effectiveness of CRA with a minimal number of therapy hours and for its application to an outpatient population. The primary new CRA procedures added in this design were Sobriety Sampling and drink-refusal training. Of great interest was the finding that marital status appeared to play a significant role in determining the effectiveness of different treatments. One potential limitation of the study was its untested generalizability to an urban population.

Examination of the Social Club Component of CRA

An additional independent study examined the Social Club component of CRA (Mallams, Godley, Hall, & Meyers, 1982). The Social Club was created primarily to provide an alcohol-free recreational environment that would be available during high-risk drinking times, such as Friday and Saturday nights. Outpatient alcoholics who already were involved in a rural treatment program were randomly assigned to one of two groups. The control group, termed Minimum Awareness ($n =$ 16), simply was informed about the Social Club and given directions on how to locate it. The experimental group, called Encouragement ($n = 19$), was privy to additional features: (1) approximately 10 contacts by a counselor, for the purpose of encouraging the subject to attend the Social Club, (2) flyers describing upcoming club events, (3) transportation to and from the club if desired, (4) membership cards, (5) problem-solving assistance from a counselor if obstacles interfered with attendance, (6) special efforts to make the subject feel comfortable whenever he attended the Social Club, and (7) attempts to provide the types of social activities preferred by the members.

With regard to attendance at the Social Club, the Encouragement group participated to a significantly greater degree than did the Minimum Awareness group, with the former group attending an average of 2.5 times during the 3-month period, and the latter group participating only 0.1 times. More importantly, the members of the Encouragement group reported an average daily alcohol consumption of 0.8 ounce, which was significantly less than that of the Minimum Awareness group's average of 3.3 ounces. The predicted group differences were noted on the Behavioral Improvement Index as well.

This study was unique in that it was the first to examine one ingredient of the CRA package: the Social Club. Furthermore, it addressed an important motivational problem faced by numerous other programs; namely, how to encourage individuals to attend potentially valuable activities. The drawbacks of the study were its small sample, a short follow-up period, and the fact that limited information was available regarding the degree of participation in the hospital's standard treatment program.

CRA with Concerned Others

A study evaluating the viability of using Community Reinforcement procedures for working with a problem drinker's Concerned Other was conducted a few years later (Sisson & Azrin 1986). All participants had contacted a community-based alcoholism treatment center in response to a family member's severe drinking problem. In this trial a distressed family member was taught a safe way to increase an uninterested problem drinker's motivation for change and treatment.

Assignments to the two groups were done randomly. The Traditional program ($n = 5$) was centered around a group education approach to alcoholism. Discussions, movies, and pamphlets focused on the disease concept of alcoholism. A behavioral technique, Systematic Encouragement, was used to foster attendance at Al-Anon meetings (Sisson & Mallams, 1981). The CRA program ($n = 7$) included the following: (1) training in awareness of alcohol problems, (2) motivational training, (3) discussions of the positive consequences for not drinking, (4) the scheduling of activities that competed with drinking, (5) the introduction of outside activities for the nondrinker, (6) training in how to respond when the problem drinker was drinking, (7) learning to allow the drinker to accept responsibility for the consequences of drinking episodes, (8) instruction in how to handle dangerous situations, and (9) increasing awareness of optimal moments for suggesting treatment to the drinker.

The results were impressive. Six of the seven drinkers whose Concerned Others were involved in the CRA group initiated treatment. In contrast, none of the Traditional group's drinkers sought treatment. With regard to drinking outcome, drinkers associated with Concerned Others in the CRA group decreased their average number of drinking days by more than half during the time that only the nondrinker was in treatment. This dropped significantly lower when the drinker entered treatment. This was not the pattern noted for drinkers whose

Concerned Other was involved in the Traditional program. Three months into treatment these individuals were still drinking nearly the same number of days per month as they had been during the baseline. The average number of drinking days each month for the Traditional group was significantly greater than that for the CRA group.

This study offered a unique approach to treating drinking problems: it initiated treatment with the nondrinker. The noteworthy outcomes were limited only by the small sample size, and the fact that the CRA therapy was a few hours longer in duration on average than was the Traditional program.

Treating Cocaine Dependency with CRA

In recent years the combination of CRA and contingency management has shown great promise in treating cocaine problems. One of the first studies was conducted with two male subjects having diagnoses of cocaine dependence according to the *Diagnostic and Statistical Manual of Mental Disorders*, third edition, revised (DSM-III-R) (Budney, Higgins, Delaney, Kent, & Bickel, 1991). And although each individual also met the criteria for marijuana dependence or abuse, neither initially expressed any interest in receiving treatment for anything other than their cocaine problem. The main intent of the study was to determine whether CRA and contingency management could increase abstinence from both cocaine and marijuana. A second interest was in ascertaining whether it was necessary for all other drug use to cease in order for the treatment of cocaine dependence to be successful. With this in mind, a multiple baseline design was employed.

During the 12-week cocaine-abstinence phase, CRA sessions were conducted twice weekly. The CRA procedures primarily included the following: (1) functional analysis of cocaine use, (2) social and recreational counseling, (3) employment counseling, (4) drug refusal-training, (5) relaxation training, and (6) reciprocal relationship counseling. The contingency management component entailed clients trading clean urine specimens for points that were redeemable for material reinforcers, such as movie tickets and dinner certificates. The number of points received was a function of the length of continuous cocaine abstinence.

During the cocaine-maintenance phase the CRA sessions were decreased to one 30-minute meeting per week. Also, the collection of urine specimens was halved, and the magnitude of the material reinforcers was reduced. This phase lasted between 3.5 and 7.5 weeks. The final phase, cocaine/marijuana abstinence, was presented to subjects as an opportunity to address their marijuana use as well. In accordance with this, reinforcements were awarded contingent upon urine specimens being negative for both cocaine and marijuana use. The duration of this phase was 12 weeks.

Cocaine abstinence increased dramatically for both subjects during the first phase of treatment, and continued throughout the maintenance phase as well. Regular marijuana use was apparent during this time, and only decreased when the cocaine/marijuana abstinence phase was introduced. Both subjects tested negative for cocaine use and positive for marijuana use at the 1- and 5- month follow-ups.

This study was important for demonstrating that a behavioral treatment package could be highly effective in addressing cocaine dependence problems. Furthermore, it offered a valuable alternative to the practice of requiring immediate cessation of all drug use prior to beginning a program, thereby potentially influencing treatment retention. But some consider this a questionable allowance, as marijuana use was apparent during several phases of the design. One should recall, however, that neither subject was particularly interested in receiving treatment for his marijuana problem in the first place. It remains to be seen in future studies whether the continued use of other drugs does indeed contribute to relapse with cocaine.

A controlled but nonrandomized study testing a CRA Plus Contingency Management treatment program similar to the one just described was conducted at approximately the same time (Higgins et al., 1991). The first 13 consecutively admitted cocaine-dependent outpatients were assigned to receive 1-hour CRA counseling sessions two times per week for a total of 12 weeks. The control group consisted of 12 of the next 15 consecutively admitted individuals with diagnoses of cocaine dependence. This second group received 12-step Standard Counseling, in which the disease model of addiction was promoted. Cocaine dependence was viewed as a disease that could be treated but not totally cured. The 12-step therapy sessions were supportive, confrontational, educational, and self-help oriented. The participants were expected to attend either 2-hour group sessions twice weekly, or a 2-hour group and 1 hour of individual therapy. Furthermore, subjects were asked to attend 1 additional self-help group per week and to identify a sponsor.

The first critical result to note is that a total of 11 out of the 13 subjects (85%) in the CRA Plus Contingency Management group completed the 12-week program, while only 5 of the 12 (42%) assigned to the Standard Counseling group did. In terms of cocaine abstinence, 10 of the CRA group members achieved 4 weeks of continuous abstinence, compared with only 3 subjects in the Standard Counseling group. Six subjects in the CRA group reached 8 weeks of abstinence, while 3 achieved 12 weeks of abstinence. None of the 12-step Standard Counseling group members even reached 8 weeks of continuous cocaine abstinence. In terms of other drug use, subjects in the CRA Plus Contingency Management group turned in a significantly greater number of urine specimens positive for marijuana. There was a trend toward showing a relationship between an individual's increased marijuana use and his decreased cocaine abstinence.

Multiple-drug dependence problems are a common occurrence among cocaine-dependent individuals, and consequently this study's inclusion of such individuals was one of its major strengths. Furthermore, the majority of the participants in the CRA group were intravenous drug users. So with regard to curtailing the transmission of AIDS alone, it is particularly noteworthy that subjects unanimously agreed to participate in the CRA program, and then evidenced a highly successful response to it. The primary limitation of the study was unknown generalizability, because all subjects were Anglo-American, and there were no crack cocaine users. Other criticisms included the reliance upon a costly incentive program, and the nonrandom subject assignment procedure. And finally, some clinicians questioned the success of a drug program in which marijuana use was still fairly common.

Next a randomized cocaine trial demonstrated that a multicomponent behavioral treatment based upon CRA Plus Contingency Management was superior to Standard Drug Counseling (Higgins et al., 1993). Therapy was divided into a 12-week primary treatment period and a 12-week aftercare segment. There were 19 subjects in each group.

As in the earlier cocaine dependence studies, subjects in the CRA group received sizable retail items and activity reinforcers for negative urine specimens during the first 12 weeks and less expensive material reinforcers the final 12 weeks. CRA procedures included the general categories of (1) relationship counseling, (2) employment counseling, (3) training in the recognition of antecedents and consequences to cocaine use, (4) drug-refusal training, (5) problem-solving training, (6) assertiveness training, and (7) recreational counseling. Additionally, willing participants who also met DSM-III-R criteria for alcohol dependence were placed on disulfiram and monitored in accordance with CRA procedures. Treatment was offered twice weekly in 1-hour counseling sessions throughout the first 12 weeks, and then once weekly during the aftercare period.

The Standard Drug Counseling group submitted urine specimens in exchange for noncontingent financial reinforcers. Therapy during each of the first 12 weeks consisted of 2 ½ hours of group and 1 hour of individual counseling based on the 12-step model of drug abuse. During weeks 13 to 24 the frequency of treatment dropped to one group or individual session per week. As a supplement to the 12-step drug counseling, participants also were (1) encouraged to attend 12-step self-help meetings, (2) assisted in identifying a self-help sponsor, and (3) instructed in relapse prevention. In addition, counselors were told that disulfiram could be used in conjunction with the regular treatment program, but only one subject was actually referred for it.

The results showed that only one CRA subject (5%) dropped out of treatment after one session, while eight (42%) of the Standard Drug Counseling subjects terminated at that time. In terms of completing the 24-week program, 58% of the subjects in the CRA group achieved this, versus 11% in the Standard Drug Counseling program. Continuous cocaine abstinence was obtained for 8 weeks by 68% of the CRA group members as compared to 11% of the comparison group. And finally, 16 weeks of continuous cocaine abstinence was realized by 42% of the CRA group, and only 5% of the Standard Drug Counseling group. Significant group differences were not detected for marijuana or alcohol use.

This first randomized trial of CRA Plus Contingency Management with cocaine-dependent individuals achieved remarkable results in all areas: agreement to begin treatment, retention in treatment, and cocaine abstinence outcome. It was limited only by questions of generalizability to crack-using, non-Anglo-American populations and by the expense of the reinforcers. The necessity for material reinforcers of this magnitude is under investigation, as is the relative contribution of the separate CRA and contingency management components.

Ongoing Controlled CRA Trials

Currently in Albuquerque, New Mexico alone there are three controlled CRA trials in progress. The projects are funded by the National Institute on Alcohol Abuse and Alcoholism (NIAAA) and the National Institute on Drug Abuse (NIDA). The grant awards were made to researchers at the University of New Mexico, both in the Psychology Department and at the Center on Alcoholism, Substance Abuse, and Addictions. The treatment programs are in various stages of data collection and analysis.

Replication and Extension of the Original CRA Outpatient Trial

The first ongoing project is a replication and extension of the original CRA outpatient trial (Azrin et al., 1982). The principal investigator for the grant is William R. Miller, and the clinical director is Robert J. Meyers. The primary purpose of the study is to determine whether CRA is superior to a standard 12-step treatment program for problem drinkers. A related interest is in ascertaining whether the addition of disulfiram to the CRA program significantly enhances treatment outcome. Furthermore, the study purports to examine the role of a subject's willingness to take disulfiram, regardless of whether he or she actually is assigned to the CRA With Disulfiram group. And finally, the design allows one to test the effectiveness of CRA within a disulfiram-ineligible sample.

The basic groups were modeled after those by Azrin et al. (1982), and were called Standard Treatment, Disulfiram Compliance, and CRA With Disulfiram. Two novel groups were added in an attempt to address the secondary research questions. A CRA Without Disulfiram group was placed in each of two tracks: one for those willing and able to take disulfiram, and one for those who were not. Subjects who were medically eligible and willing to take disulfiram were assigned randomly to one of four groups in the first track: Standard Treatment with Disulfiram, Disulfiram Compliance, CRA With Disulfiram, or CRA Without Disulfiram. Individuals who were unwilling or unable to take disulfiram were randomly placed in one of two groups in the second track: Standard Treatment without Disulfiram or CRA Without Disulfiram. The goal was to recruit 40 subjects per group. The full design is represented in Figure 1.1 at the top of the next page.

Group A, Standard Treatment With Disulfiram, was based on the disease model of alcoholism and was conducted by two nondegreed counselors who had 15 and 18 years of experience in the field of alcoholism treatment. The core of these procedures included (1) encouragement to attend AA meetings, a schedule of AA meetings, and information as to which meetings would be most beneficial; (2) discussions of AA literature, including the 12 steps and traditions of AA; (3) prompts to obtain an AA sponsor; (4) an explanation of R. A. Jellinek's (1952) description of gamma alcoholism; (5) a viewing of the Father Martin film *Chalk Talk*; (6) encouragement to attend an evening recovery group facilitated by one of the Group A therapists; and (7) arrangements to take disulfiram according to the rules of the Center on Alcoholism, Substance Abuse, and Addictions. This entailed attending a lecture on disulfiram and receiving a physical examination from the center's medical staff. Disulfiram was administered in 500-mg doses twice weekly by the LPN on duty.

Subjects assigned to Group B, Disulfiram Compliance, received the same basic treatment as those in Group A. In addition, however, they were trained in the CRA disulfiram compliance procedure. This procedure required that clients bring a Concerned Other to their intake session, so that he or she could be instructed in how to monitor and reinforce the taking of disulfiram. Positive communication skills were taught as part of this procedure, in order to increase the chances

INITIAL SCREENING

Medically Eligible and Willing to Take Disulfiram?
[Nonrandom assignment]

	YES			NO	
	[random assignment]			[random assignment]	
Group A	Group B	Group C	Group D	Group E	Group F
Standard Treatment With Disulfiram	Disulfiram Compliance	CRA With Disulfiram	CRA Without Disulfiram	Standard Treatment Without Disulfiram	CRA Without Disulfiram

FIGURE 1.1. Research design for a replication and extension of the original CRA outpatient trial (principal investigator was William R. Miller).

that the drinker would cooperate in taking the disulfiram. As a final measure, the monitor was instructed to contact the therapist if the drinker refused the disulfiram 2 days in a row.

Group C, CRA With Disulfiram, received the disulfiram compliance procedure just described for Group B, as well as the complete CRA treatment. The CRA components included (1) Sobriety Sampling, (2) a functional analysis, (3) problem-solving training, (4) social skills training, (5) social or recreational counseling, and (6) mood monitoring. When deemed necessary, additional CRA procedures were utilized as well: (7) behavioral marital therapy, (8) reinforcer access counseling, (9) job-finding counseling, (10) relaxation training, and (11) drink-refusal training. Subjects in Group D, CRA Without Disulfiram, received the same CRA treatment as Group C, except that disulfiram was neither prescribed nor recommended.

The second track, which was reserved for those who were unwilling or unable to take disulfiram, was composed of two groups. Group E, Standard Treatment Without Disulfiram, involved a program identical to that of Group A, with the exception that disulfiram was not prescribed. Group F, CRA Without Disulfiram, was the same treatment as that provided to members of Group D.

Treatment sessions were scheduled weekly in all groups. Additional sessions were left to the discretion of therapists. Follow-up interviews for all subjects were conducted at 2, 3, 4, 6, 9, 12, 18, and 24 months following intake.

The final sample comprised 238 clients: 83% male, 55% Hispanic, 39% white, non-Hispanic, 4% Native American, and 2% from other racial or ethnic backgrounds. The data on this project are in the process of being statistically analyzed.

CRA with Heroin Abusers

Another trial underway at the University of New Mexico is a study designed to test the efficacy of CRA with a heroin-abusing population. The principal investigator of the grant is Patrick Abbott, and the clinical director is Robert J. Meyers. The main purpose of this experiment is to contrast CRA with a standard treatment package for heroin-dependent individuals. A second interest is to test the potential benefit of adding a specific relapse prevention component to the CRA program.

Eligible subjects were randomly assigned to one of three groups: CRA + Methadone, CRA + Methadone + Relapse Prevention, or Standard Counseling + Methadone. So regardless of the group assignment, all subjects received methadone daily in accordance with the *Federal Register*'s 1989 Guidelines for methadone maintenance. Individuals were eligible for take-home privileges after 90 days, but then only if they complied with the program's policies and procedures.

In addition to methadone maintenance therapy, subjects in Group A received the following CRA procedures: (1) a CRA induction, (2) a CRA functional analysis, (3) Sobriety Sampling, (4) problem-solving training, (5) drug-refusal training, (6) communication skills training, (7) behavioral marital therapy, (8) reinforcer access counseling, (9) social and recreational counseling, and (10) a Job Finding Club. Fourteen individual sessions were scheduled at the rate of one per week.

Subjects assigned to Group B received methadone, the full CRA program, and 6 sessions that targeted relapse prevention. These additional sessions focused on 3 primary areas: (1) skills building, (2) cognitive restructuring, and (3) the balancing of lifestyle (Marlatt & Gordon, 1985). Sample topics included controlling urges, generating alternative cognitive responses, coping with high-risk situations, developing an emergency plan, finding "alternative highs," and dealing with the Abstinence Violation Effect (Marlatt & Gordon, 1985). Group C subjects received methadone and a standard treatment program that primarily provided supportive counseling and referrals for social needs. The emphasis was on concrete services and solutions to immediate problems. The 3 basic phases included (1) problem identification, (2) problem-solving activities, and (3) the monitoring of clients' progress. Individualized treatment plans were devised for each subject. A total of 14 individual weekly sessions were scheduled in order to allow problem-solving time for the identified issues.

Follow-up assessments were conducted at 1, 3, 6, 9, 12, and 18 months after intake. Statistical analyses currently are being conducted.

CRA with a Homeless Population

A third research project in progress at the University of New Mexico is an application of CRA with an alcohol-abusing or -dependent homeless population. The program is under the direction of the principal investigator, Jane Ellen Smith, and the clinical director, Robert J. Meyers. The main purpose of the study is to contrast a homeless shelter's standard treatment with a CRA program. The contribution of the disulfiram component to the overall effectiveness of the CRA program also is being examined. A third interest of the study is in determining the effect of simply being willing and able to take disulfiram, regardless of whether one actually is assigned to that particular group. The design of the study is outlined in Figure 1.2.

As noted above, individuals were asked whether or not they would be willing to take disulfiram if they happened to be randomly assigned to that group. Those willing and medically able to take disulfiram were marked for Track 1, while subjects unwilling or unable to take disulfiram were placed in Track 2. Track 1 consisted of 3 groups. The Standard Treatment group (STD) consisted of a homeless shelter's basic program. Components included (1) access to on-site AA meetings 4 days a week, (2) an available substance abuse counselor with a 12-step orientation, (3) a job program that assisted with temporary employment, (4) income management assistance, (5) free breakfasts, (6) access to showers, (7) a clothing exchange, (8) telephones, (9) mail service, and (10) storage. The shelter was open weekdays from 8:00 A.M. to 2:00 P.M.

Participants in the second group in Track 1, CRA With Disulfiram (CRA + D), were able to take advantage of all the services regularly available through the homeless shelter. In addition, CRA group therapy sessions were held 5 days a week. The groups included (1) a Job Finding Club, (2) problem-solving training, (3) drink-refusal training, (4) independent living skills instruction, (5) Social Club, and (6) community meetings. Two prizes were awarded weekly for group attendance. When relevant, subjects and their Concerned Other received behavioral marital therapy. Typically, subjects also attended an average of 5 individual therapy sessions over the course of the 3-month treatment phase. These sessions dealt primarily with basic case management issues. And finally, all subjects in the CRA + D group were given a pre-

INITIAL SCREENING

Medically Able and Willing to Take Disulfiram?
[Nonrandom assignment]

YES	NO
Track 1 [random assignment]	Track 2 [random assignment]

Group STD	Group CRA + D	Group CRA - D	Group STD	Group CRA - D
Standard Treatment	CRA With Disulfiram	CRA Without Disulfiram	Standard Treatment	CRA Without Disulfiram

FIGURE 1.2. Research design for CRA trial with a homeless population (principal investigator was Jane Ellen Smith; co-principal investigator was Robert J. Meyers). For a description of each group, see text.

scription for disulfiram. Since many of these individuals did not have a Concerned Other available to assist with the disulfiram compliance procedure, all attended a daily group meeting in which the project nurse dispensed their disulfiram and served as the monitor. The third group in Track 1 was CRA Without Disulfiram (CRA - D). The treatment protocol for this group was identical to that of CRA + D, except for the fact that subjects were not prescribed disulfiram and did not attend a daily disulfiram compliance group.

Track 2 was designed to accommodate individuals who were either unwilling or unable to take disulfiram. There were two groups in Track 2: Standard Treatment and CRA Without Disulfiram. The subjects in these groups received the same treatment protocols as their comparable groups in Track 1. Again, duplicate groups were included to ascertain whether subjects' mere willingness or ability to take disulfiram affected treatment outcome.

All subjects in both tracks were provided with 12 weeks of housing by the project. Random Breathalyzer tests were conducted at these premises on a regular basis, and subjects were sent for urine samples periodically. Any infraction of housing rules, such as the use of alcohol or drugs, threats of violence, or thefts resulted in the loss of housing privileges for a designated period of time. Return to housing was based on compliance.

Follow-ups were conducted at 2, 4, 6, 9, and 12 months after intake. Statistical analyses for this study are underway.

Sharing the Wealth

This book is an outgrowth of work done with the Community Reinforcement Approach over the last 17 years. During this time there have been scientific articles reporting the efficacy of CRA trials, and reviews describing CRA as one of the more effective treatments for alcohol abusers (Miller, Brown, et al., 1995). Yet, until now, no one has explained exactly how to implement the CRA program. The remaining chapters of this book are based on our experience using CRA in clinical research trials and in clinical practice. It is our special blend of CRA philosophy and procedures set forth in a "cookbook" package for therapists.

2

CRA Assessment

The CRA assessment process consists of three main components: identifying and enhancing motivation for change, gathering background and basic substance-use information, and conducting the CRA Functional Analysis. The information obtained in this early stage of therapy is utilized in subsequent sessions to formulate a treatment plan and to monitor progress.

IDENTIFYING AND ENHANCING MOTIVATION

One of the basic premises of CRA is that people will be motivated to change their substance-abusing behavior if they are reinforced (rewarded) in so doing. To facilitate this process, considerable attention is devoted throughout the course of therapy to identifying a client's "reinforcers." A positive reinforcer is any object or behavior whose presentation increases the rate of the behavior it follows. Although there are a number of fairly universal reinforcers, one cannot assume that a compliment or a kind act will be interpreted as a reinforcer by everyone. Consequently, it is necessary to discover each client's own unique reinforcers, particularly those strong enough to increase the rate of sober behavior. Take, for example, the drinker who cherishes the time he spends with his son, but who is only permitted to do so by his ex-wife when he is sober. If he increases the amount of time he is sober in an effort to see his son more, the time spent with his son would be considered a powerful reinforcer.

The identification of an individual's reinforcers begins during the assessment phase by noting the source of the client's motivation for seeking treatment in the first place. In other words, is the individual requesting therapy because of a desire to introduce healthy changes into his or her life? Or does the client's current interest in addressing an alcohol problem stem from external pressures from a spouse, boss, or probation officer? Regardless of whether the client wants to increase sober behavior in order to receive something pleasant (positive reinforcer) or avoid something aversive (negative reinforcer), the therapist's job is to make these reinforcers salient. Reference to these motivators may prove useful if the client appears to need a reminder about the specific reasons for investing energy into changing problematic behaviors.

There are several additional ways by which CRA attempts to enhance motivation during the initial assessment. One entails conducting the first session as soon as possible once the request for an appointment has been received. Motivation appears to be particularly high at this point, frequently because of an alcohol-related crisis that has elicited a tremendous amount of fear or pain. But since a client's motivation often dwindles with the fading of a crisis, time is of the essence. For this reason it is also common to hold several meetings in close succession at the start of treatment.

The next way in which CRA enhances motivation is by setting positive expectations about treatment outcome. In part, this means approaching the entire treatment process with a positive attitude that is respectful of a client's defenses. It includes avoiding value-laden labels by speaking in terms of an individual's alcohol-related "problems," instead of referring to the person as an "alcoholic." Setting positive treatment expectations also involves pointing out the negative consequences of drinking while conveying the message that there are achievable solutions to these problems. And finally, it entails beginning to demonstrate how CRA can help a client obtain the things that are reinforcing to him or her.

The last way in which CRA addresses motivational issues during the assessment phase is by including a Concerned Other in the process. Typically this individual is highly invested in seeing the client change his or her alcohol consumption patterns. With some training the Concerned Other can learn how to express feelings appropriately and how to offer support in a manner that is reinforcing and motivating for the client. (Refer to Chapter 9: CRA Marital Therapy, for a complete description of the Concerned Other's multifaceted role in the therapy process.)

BACKGROUND AND SUBSTANCE USE INFORMATION

It is advisable to conduct your own intakes whenever possible. This both spares the client from having to relate his or her story several times, and allows you to probe for details that may be valuable for the therapeutic process. In terms of the types of information to collect, CRA recommends that you cover at least the following topics: presenting problem(s), quantity and frequency of alcohol and other drug use, background information in several areas (medical, psychological, legal, marital, familial, occupational), alcohol-related problems in each of these domains, and motivation for change.

There are standardized psychological instruments available to assist in the gathering of this information. (For a complete review see Miller, Westerberg, & Waldron, 1995.) The tools vary in complexity and administration time, and consequently you must determine your own individual needs and constraints. For instance, there are relatively lengthy comprehensive instruments that address both substance use and other life problems. Examples include the Addiction Severity Index (McLellan, Luborsky, Woody, & O'Brien, 1980) and the Brief Drinker Profile (Miller & Marlatt, 1987). There are straightforward procedures for collecting data on the quantity and frequency of alcohol consumption (Cahalan, Cisin, & Crossley, 1969), and specialized instruments that target alcohol-related problems (the Drinker Inventory of Consequences; Miller, Tonigan, & Longabaugh, 1994). And finally, there are questionnaires to measure motivation to change, such as the University of Rhode Island Change Instrument (Prochaska & DiClemente, 1986), and the Stages of Change Readiness and Treatment Eagerness Scale (Miller, 1993). Regardless of the assessment instruments selected, keep in mind when interpreting the results to the client that the goal is not to use this information to "break down denial," but rather to motivate the individual to make positive behavior changes.

If the client's Concerned Other is present at the first session, you may elect to interview him or her while the client is completing the pencil-and-paper questionnaires. As noted earlier, this individual may prove to be an essential player in the client's treatment plan, and consequently it is helpful to develop an alliance early in therapy. Enlisting this person's support entails showing empathy for the effect the client's drinking has had on him or her, and then identifying the Concerned Other's reinforcers as well. It is important, however, not to assume that this individual is substance free. In fact, if you suspect that this person also has a substance abuse problem, it is best to ask the individual to complete the assessment instruments immediately. In either event, you should have the Concerned Other present during a description of CRA and its rationale.

CRA FUNCTIONAL ANALYSIS

Description and Objectives

Today most inpatient and many outpatient alcohol treatment programs still are built around the concept of denial, and the belief that denial must be handled with confrontation. The message of the confrontational approach is clear: "You're an alcoholic and you can never drink again." One of the notions underlying CRA is that it is more useful to approach the problem from a different angle, and instead to ask: Why exactly is this person drinking? What are the reinforcement systems? It recognizes that from a client's perspective the drinking behavior can be viewed as adaptive. That is, it performs a survival function, by masking anxiety or depression, or by camouflaging a marital situation in which there is no emotional or sexual intimacy. CRA works directly to address those problem areas. The basic assessment tool used to begin this entire process is the functional analysis.

A functional analysis is a structured interview that examines the antecedents and consequences of a specific behavior of interest, such as the consumption of alcohol. The first purpose of a functional analysis is to outline each individual client's triggers for drinking behavior; to designate the chain of events that leads to drinking. This is a critical step in treatment because many individuals with alcohol problems believe that drinking "just happens." The client's recognition that drinking episodes are the result of many small decisions is an important part of relapse prevention. The second purpose of a functional analysis is to clarify the consequences of a behavior. Again, each client's history is reviewed in an attempt to specify both the immediate and long-term results of the drinking behavior.

The CRA Functional Analysis plays a prominent role in arranging an ongoing positive, reinforcing environment for a client that encourages sobriety. One segment of it identifies past, current, and potential future positive reinforcers in major areas of the client's life, including relationships, job, and recreational activities. These positive reinforcers are situations or events that increase the likelihood that sober behavior will be repeated. CRA attempts "to rearrange the vocational, family and social reinforcers of the alcoholic such that a time-out from these reinforcers would occur if he began to drink" (Hunt & Azrin,

1973, p. 93). In essence, it is a comprehensive approach that examines the total person in the context of environment and looks for reinforcers that support sobriety.

Identifying Antecedents to Drinking

Traditional functional analyses explore antecedents or "triggers" to drinking. These are thoughts, feelings, or behaviors that precede a drinking episode and that are instrumental in leading the individual to drink. The first section of the CRA Functional Analysis also examines these triggers and the associated high-risk situations (see Appendix 2.A).

Explore with your client the chain of events that sets him or her up to drink. Ask the client to give you an example of a common type of drinking episode. In this way fairly specific questions can be posed regarding the event, but the responses will tend to have broad applicability. First ask specific questions about *external* triggers:

1. *"Who* are you usually with when you drink?" A certain friend or relative may be a trigger to drink. Look for responses such as, "I don't know. Well, lots of times when I hang out with Harold I guess we end up drinking." The client may not have realized that such a direct connection between Harold and alcohol existed.

2. *"Where* do you usually drink?" Often the client will say, "Well, I went to a bar with a friend, but I meant to drink only a soda." This is the therapist's opportunity to start pointing out high-risk environments.

3. *"When* do you usually drink?" Are there certain days? Times of the day? The client may discover, for example, that the excessive drinking tends to occur on the two evenings that he or she attends night classes after working all day.

Next, ask the client specific questions about *internal* triggers for drinking:

1. "What are you usually *thinking* about right before you drink?" Encourage the client to report as many thoughts as can be remembered. It would be important to discover whether the client had such ideas as, "I worked hard today and I deserve a beer." Outlining the thinking process is critical, since the client needs to see that at some point he or she makes a decision to drink; that it is not an automatic process. Thoughts also supply information about the client's defense system. For example, does the client utilize rationalization or projection? And finally, the thoughts provide valuable insight into the feelings that were associated with drinking.

2. "What are you usually *feeling physically* right before you drink?" With some prompting, clients can focus in on bodily sensations that may suggest various states of arousal. For example, a pounding head and a clenched jaw may imply that the client is angry, while a knot in the stomach and sweaty hands may represent an anxiety response.

3. "What are you usually *feeling emotionally* right before you drink?" Clients often are unaware of this at first, and consequently need to be trained to recognize and then label their feelings. You would want to know, for instance, if the client was drinking in response to anger, frustration, or despair. If a client has not learned how to deal with these emotions more adaptively, he or she may rely on the more familiar escape response: drinking.

What follows is an example of a therapist beginning a CRA Functional Analysis with a client. This first section illustrates how you would explain the purpose of the analysis and link the relevant assessment information already collected. It then shows how antecedents to drinking would be outlined and entered onto a chart in columns labeled for external and internal triggers. Note that the first functional analysis chart will be completed for the client's most common drinking episode.

THERAPIST: Another thing we need to do today, Bud, is to take a look at the kinds of problems drinking has caused you in the past. According to the assessment information it looks like drinking has at least caused you some legal problems. What other kinds of problems do *you* think it has created?

CLIENT: Well, I did get my second DWI, and Gloria is upset with me, but my lawyer says it isn't going to be a big problem.

THERAPIST: But your assessment materials state that your wife actually left you once because of your drinking.

Note: It is important to be familiar with the client's assessment information, for it can be used to show the client that you fully understand the severity of the drinking problem. You would not utilize this information to confront the client, but rather to motivate him to accept treatment.

CLIENT: I guess it has caused me some hassles, but I know lots of people who drink more than I do.

THERAPIST: Well, I'm sure that's right. But what we're going to do today is take a look at your drinking behavior through a process called a functional analysis. We need to get a good clear picture of the types of problems drinking has caused you specifically, and the things that lead you to drink in the first place. We'll start by looking at some of the things in your environment that always seem to be a part of your drinking episodes, and then some of the things going on inside of you at those times.

CLIENT: What do you mean? I drink just because I like to drink.

THERAPIST: OK, but let's see if we can come up with some understanding of why you drink to the extent that it causes you problems. The first thing we need to look at are what we call "triggers" for drinking. Triggers can be situations, thoughts, feelings, behaviors, or even people that seem to lead up to a drinking episode. For example, I had a client once who always went out and drank after an argument with his wife. So the argument with his wife would trigger the drinking episode.

CLIENT: Oh, I see what you mean. Every time my old buddy Jack comes into town, we end up staying out most of the night drinking.

THERAPIST: That's right, Bud. Jack would be an example of a person who's a trigger for you to drink. You seem to understand the idea of looking for triggers. Let's go through this systematically now.

Note: At this point you would either go to the blackboard to illustrate the functional analysis, or hand the client a chart similar to the one in Appendix 2.A.

THERAPIST: Let's start by breaking down the triggers, the things that lead up to drinking, into several categories. We'll look at external triggers, or things in your environment first. Now you mentioned that your buddy, Jack, was a trigger for your drinking. How often do you see Jack?

CLIENT: Usually only about once a month. But every time I see him we sure tie a load on.

THERAPIST: Well, how about we start off by looking at the people you drink with on a more regular basis? Let's look at your chart. The first question asks, "Who are you *usually* with when you drink?"

CLIENT: About three days a week I head out to the Exchange after work with some guys from the office, and then on Sunday afternoon I go over to my brother's house to watch a game on TV. We drink most of the afternoon there.

THERAPIST: OK. Let's look at these as two different examples of common drinking occasions. How about we start with your weekday drinking, since this happens more often?

CLIENT: Sounds OK to me.

Note: A functional analysis chart is completed for several representative common types of drinking episodes. You probably would want to group together highly similar incidents. For example, the therapist here will treat the weekday drinking that occurs in the same bar with the same people as one type of episode, and the Sunday afternoon drinking as a second one.

THERAPIST: Great. So who do you drink with after work those three week-days?

CLIENT: I usually go with Fred and Bill.

THERAPIST: OK. So I'll put their names here right on the chart in the first column. And you'll see that we already have the answers to the next two questions, because we know *where* and *when* you usually drink. I'll fill them in, too.

Note: Refer now to Appendix 2.B for the completed chart.

THERAPIST: So when you first decide to go to the Exchange, what's on your mind? Did you guys have a bad day at work? Do you just not want to go home? What's the deal?

CLIENT: Well, I thought I just went to have a couple of beers and a few laughs. But now you're making it sound like I have a big problem.

THERAPIST: Remember that we're just trying to figure out the reasons why you drink.

CLIENT: All right. By the time 5 o'clock rolls around I'm just tired of the bull.

THERAPIST: What do you mean by that?

CLIENT: My boss is always on my back. He really pisses me off. I need to get out and blow off steam, I guess.

THERAPIST: Sounds like you're talking about what we call internal triggers. So let's look at the chart again and see if we can answer the questions in the second column. These are harder, because they have to do with things going on inside of you. The first question asks, "What are you usually thinking about right before you drink?"

CLIENT: I'm thinking about how much I can't stand my boss.

THERAPIST: Why does your boss tick you off so much?

CLIENT: I just don't think he treats me fair. I see how he treats others.

THERAPIST: Let's put these thoughts down. OK. You say he treats you unfairly. How does that make you feel?

CLIENT: My boss really makes me mad, and he makes me feel like I'm not doing a good job.

THERAPIST: OK. So he makes you feel mad. Are you also saying he makes you feel inadequate?

CLIENT: Yes, and embarrassed.

THERAPIST: Let's add these feelings to the chart then under question #3. Now, when you're feeling really angry, do you ever notice any physical sensations?

CLIENT: Yeah. Sometimes I'm so upset that I start to shake.

THERAPIST: I'm putting that back here, then, for question #2: physical feelings.

Note: The therapist has now completed the set of internal triggers on the chart. A brief summary of the triggers follows.

THERAPIST: From what you've said, Bud, you head out to drink with your friends several nights a week after work because you're angry and upset about how your boss has treated you. You also feel embarrassed and inadequate. What we're eventually going to do is come up with some other ways of dealing with these feelings so that you don't always have to turn to alcohol.

The Drinking Behavior

At this point it is important to move directly from the triggers for drinking to the drinking behavior itself. This serves to impress upon the client in yet another way this crucial connection. It also is an opportune time to gather explicit details on the drinking pattern.

What follows is a continuation of the conversation between the client, Bud, and his therapist. Recall that the antecedents to drinking already have been covered.

THERAPIST: Now that we have a clear understanding of what leads you to drink certain weeknights after work, let's discuss in more detail the drinking itself. The first questions under the "Behavior" column ask, "What do you usually drink, and how much?"

CLIENT: I usually have a couple of beers.

THERAPIST: When you say "a couple of beers," do you mean a couple of cans? Pitchers? What exactly do you mean?

CLIENT: I drink about 5 to 6 12-ounce bottles of Miller.

THERAPIST: How long does it take you to drink those 5 to 6 beers?

CLIENT: We usually get there about 6 o'clock, and we leave between 8 and 8:30.

THERAPIST: I'm going to fill in the chart then.

Note: Refer to Appendix 2.B. This information should be as specific as possible.

Short-Term Positive Consequences of Drinking

With most alcohol-abusing clients, drinking eventually leads to negative consequences. However, upon first drinking alcohol, most clients do experience some short-term positive effects. Alcohol initially may reduce anxiety, help a client feel more comfortable socializing, or assist a client in temporarily forgetting his or her problems. It is important for you to acknowledge these positive effects, but to then point out the fact that these benefits are always short lived. Additionally, you might discuss how the initial positive effects of alcohol may not be "worth" the inevitable negative consequences.

The dialogue between Bud and the therapist now reviews the short-term positive consequences of drinking. Note how the therapist continues to convey a positive attitude. Part of this entails looking for opportunities to reinforce the client.

THERAPIST: Bud, you told me earlier that you drank simply because you like to drink. Can you tell me what you mean by that?

CLIENT: I just like the taste of beer. And when I'm drinking I don't seem to worry about my problems.

THERAPIST: OK. Let's look at the fourth column on your chart now. So you're saying that you enjoy drinking because of the taste. I'll put that under #5, "physical feelings." You're also saying that you don't worry about your problems when you're drinking. I'll put that under #6, "emotional feelings," since it implies that you're less troubled and feel more relaxed. I guess we really could place "it's relaxing" under "physical feelings," too.

CLIENT: I never thought of it in those terms, but I'm not going to argue with you.

THERAPIST: Can you identify any of the pleasant thoughts you have when you're out drinking with the guys?

CLIENT: I don't know. How about, "I'm not a bad guy. The boss is just a jerk"?

THERAPIST: Good. That goes under #4. What do you think it is about drinking with Fred and Bill that you really enjoy?

CLIENT: They hate the boss as much as I do. We sit around and make fun of him together.

THERAPIST: OK. Is there anything special about why you always go to the Exchange?

CLIENT: Not really. It's just close to work.

THERAPIST: Fine. Anything special about drinking *after work*?

CLIENT: It's a good time to unwind.

THERAPIST: I'm putting these on the chart for questions #1, #2, and #3 under "Short-Term Positive Consequences." You know, Bud, you really seem to be getting the hang of this. I appreciate the fact that you're working so hard with me.

Note: The therapist took an opportunity to reinforce the client for his hard work and effort. This tactic is in line with the CRA philosophy of staying positive and keeping the client motivated. One should note that the functional analysis thus far has served to lay the groundwork for showing the client the long-term negative consequences that result from his drinking behavior just outlined.

Identifying Negative Consequences of Drinking

As already stated, in order to do a good functional analysis you must be very familiar with all of the client's assessment information. A clear profile of the client's history is essential, particularly since many clients minimize the negative consequences of excessive alcohol consumption.

The therapist and Bud now discuss the negative consequences of, or the problems associated with, his drinking. The therapist carefully covers all of the common problem areas and enters the information on the functional analysis chart. While completing this last column, the therapist will check to be certain that the client clearly sees the connection between his drinking and the list of adverse consequences. In the event that he does not, the matter will be pursued further.

THERAPIST: The last part of the functional analysis involves taking a look at the negative things that have happened to you because of your drinking. Today we'll just list some of these negative consequences, and later we'll start figuring out ways to change the behaviors that bring on these consequences. For instance, let's first talk about the legal problems you've had to face recently because of your drinking.

CLIENT: Well, like I told you before, I'm here because I got a second DWI.

My lawyer said it would look good for me to get into a program.

THERAPIST: Do you feel that this is a problem? Do you see that there is a connection between your legal problems and the drinking that you do with your friends after work?

CLIENT: Well, I guess so. I did get both DWIs on my way home from the Exchange.

THERAPIST: OK. I'm going to list this under legal problems. What other problems has your drinking at the Exchange caused you?

CLIENT: You mean like when I get home late and Gloria is mad at me because I've missed dinner?

THERAPIST: Yes, that's a good example. Can you think of any other people you've had problems with because of your drinking?

CLIENT: I got into an argument one night at the bar, and a glass got smashed on my hand. I ended up missing work the next day because I had to get stitches. My wife sat there in the Emergency Room, so she missed work that day, too.

THERAPIST: Let's see how we can fit these into our last column: "Long-Term Negative Consequences." So you're having interpersonal problems with your wife at times, and physically you even got hurt one night. It sounds like it created a job problem, because you missed work. I bet that had financial repercussions, too.

CLIENT: Yes, I found out that my health insurance wouldn't even cover the hospital visit because we hadn't met our deductible yet. And my wife probably will lose her wages for the time she missed.

THERAPIST: What about any emotional problems created by your weeknight drinking?

CLIENT: Well, Gloria is always upset when I get home late those evenings, and I guess that kind of upsets me, too, then.

THERAPIST: OK. So you can see where I'm charting that. Bud, now that we've gone through a complete analysis of your weeknight drinking, can you see a connection between some of your problems and your drinking?

Note: If the client saw the connection between his drinking and the negative consequences, then the therapist would proceed with a functional analysis for the second type of drinking episode: Sunday afternoons at his brother's. However, if the client was unable to see the connection between his drinking and the negative consequences, then the therapist would have to continue working with the client until this association was made. An example of this latter case follows:

THERAPIST: I'm a little confused here, Bud. Why don't you help me out. You're here because of a DWI, right? Would you be willing to say that your drinking has at least caused you some legal hassles?

CLIENT: OK, well I'm one of the unlucky ones who got caught. Everybody drinks and drives.

THERAPIST: Help me out again. Didn't we just spend the last half hour talking about all of the negative things that have happened to you because of your late nights out at the Exchange? Didn't we just list interpersonal, physical, emotional, and financial problems that seemed related to your drinking?

CLIENT: OK. I guess I understand what you're getting at here. But I know for a fact that my brother has even *more* problems from his drinking.

THERAPIST: You may be right. But I'm concerned now with the problems that *you're* facing because of your drinking.

Note: The CRA therapist simply relied on the assessment information, including the functional analysis, to present the picture to the client. The therapist used the factual details just provided by the client himself.

Positive Triggers for Nondrinking Behavior

All too often treatment programs try to focus solely on these negative consequences as a way of motivating the client to change. However, experience tells us that most people do not change as a result of therapists emphasizing only negative consequences. These clients typically have had *many* people constantly pointing out to them the problems attributable to their excessive alcohol consumption, and unfortunately it has not worked as an effective intervention. CRA's Functional Analysis goes beyond using just the negative consequences to motivate the drinker to change.

This second phase of the functional analysis is one of CRA's most important contributions to the field. It begins again with an exploration of triggers, but this time the antecedents are for *non*drinking behavior. The purpose of this analysis is to demonstrate to the client that he or she already takes pleasure in certain activities that do not involve alcohol, and that a number of positive benefits are associated with these activities. Later you would encourage the client to add more of these nondrinking behaviors or new ones to the daily schedule.

Note that the format for this functional analysis is modeled after the one already introduced for drinking behaviors. A separate chart is provided (see Appendix 2.C).

The therapist now presents to the client the notion of a second functional analysis, but this time for specific, pleasurable, nondrinking behaviors. An example of one representative activity will be charted.

THERAPIST: OK, Bud, we're going to switch gears now, so that we can look at some of the positive activities in your life that aren't associated with alcohol. One of the things we do with CRA is try to help you increase the things in your life that are positive, the things that make you happy. What's one thing that you really enjoy doing that *doesn't involve alcohol*?

CLIENT: I suppose riding my bicycle.

THERAPIST: That's great. Now let's take this activity and see if we can fit it into this second chart, one that deals with enjoyable nondrinking activities. Why don't you tell me a little about your riding?

CLIENT: Well, I usually ride by myself two afternoons a week, and some Saturday mornings I go with a friend or two.

THERAPIST: So you ride by yourself twice a week, and then periodically with friends on Saturday. Let's look at these as two different types of riding. How about we begin with the most common event, the weekday riding by yourself?

CLIENT: Sure. What do you want to know?

THERAPIST: When and where do you typically ride?

CLIENT: It depends on when I leave work and whether I stop at the Exchange. If I head straight home on time I see other cyclists on the main road, and it makes me want to go for a ride there myself.

THERAPIST: Let's go back to our chart and plug in this information under "External Triggers." It looks like you ride near your home, and you do it right after work if you get out on time and head straight home. Seeing other cyclists puts you in the mood to ride.

CLIENT: That's right.

THERAPIST: Now let's look at the *internal* triggers. What are you thinking about before you ride, and what do you feel emotionally and physically?

CLIENT: Well, I usually feel excited or happy when I think about it. I guess I'm looking forward to it because it's going to help me relax. I can even feel my body get less tense, calmer, when I think about riding.

THERAPIST: Sounds good. I've listed these on the chart. Now the next category is already mostly answered. Under "Behavior" we can list riding for question #1, and two weekday afternoons for question #2. What should we put for the third question?

CLIENT: It takes about an hour.

Note: Refer to the completed chart (Appendix 2.D).

Identifying the Negative Consequences of Nondrinking Behavior

Many interesting and enjoyable activities frequently have an unpleasant component as well. Often this negative side of the activity is more immediate than the positive aspects. And although the negative effects typically are brief in duration, nevertheless, at times, they serve to deter the client from engaging in the nondrinking activity altogether. Consequently you should acknowledge the existence of the negative consequences before moving to the positive. At a later point you may even use a problem-solving strategy to eliminate some of these negative components (see Chapter 6). The dialogue continues.

THERAPIST: Riding your bike is a great activity and it has numerous positive effects. But is there any part of your riding that you dislike? Do you sometimes find yourself making excuses so that you don't have to go?

CLIENT: What do you mean?

THERAPIST: Do you ever ride even though you're not really excited about it? Or maybe it would help to remember a time when you were thinking about riding, but then you talked yourself into going for a drink instead.

CLIENT: If I'm already exhausted it's harder to get myself to go for a ride. But I usually push myself if I haven't gotten out much that week. Oh, I think I see what you mean.

THERAPIST: Great. Let's go back to the chart now and answer the questions in the column labeled "Short-Term Negative Consequences." The first question has to do with disliking something about who you ride with. You said you actually ride alone on these days. Is there anything unpleasant about riding alone?

CLIENT: Once in a while I'd rather have someone along to shoot the bull with. Usually I don't mind. But you know, I bet I do focus on my aches and pains more since I don't have anyone to distract me.

THERAPIST: Good. Question #2 asks what you dislike about *where* you ride.

CLIENT: Well, sometimes the traffic is heavy and I feel like I'm going to get run off the road. I guess I get mad at the drivers at times.

THERAPIST: That's perfect. I'm going to fill in "gets mad" under question #6 since it asks about feelings. How about question #3? What do you dislike about *when* you ride?

CLIENT: It's the traffic problem again. There seems to be more right after work, since people are heading home. Oh, and sometimes I have to hurry before it gets dark, and I don't stretch enough first. It makes me sore the next day.

THERAPIST: I'll put that part under question #5 about physical feelings. Earlier you were saying something about feeling really tired. I'll jot that down, too. What about question #4? Any unpleasant thoughts?

CLIENT: Sometimes I feel a little rushed because of something I have to do that night. But I can't think of unpleasant thoughts, unless you mean, "I better hurry or I'll be late."

THERAPIST: That's fine, Bud. You've done a great job.

Note: Since CRA is a positive approach, do not feel obligated to push the client too hard to establish negative consequences. As mentioned earlier, at a later point you might even spend time helping the client find ways to eliminate some of the short-term negative aspects.

Identifying the Positive Consequences of Nondrinking Behavior

CRA is based on the learning theory belief that maladaptive behavior has been learned and consequently can be "unlearned." Healthy, appropriate behaviors can be substituted instead. To facilitate this process, motivate the client by helping identify positive reinforcers associated with these appropriate behaviors. This could be followed later by guidance regarding how to actually engage in these behaviors more often.

The final segment of this dialogue illustrates how to help the client identify all of the positive consequences of his nondrinking activity.

THERAPIST: You're doing a fine job, Bud. Let's now continue with the last category: "Long-Term Positive Consequences." That one should be easy for you. Go ahead and start at the top, and let's work our way down.

CLIENT: I feel better when I ride, so I'd say my relationship with Gloria is smoother. I blow off steam on my bike, so I don't complain as much to her about my job. Is that what you're looking for?

THERAPIST: Yes, exactly. Keep going. I'll help you if you get stuck.

CLIENT: Well, riding keeps my weight down, and it's good for my blood pressure. I've already said it helps me reduce stress and feel better. I can't think of any legal benefits. And I'm not so sure about how it helps my job.

THERAPIST: Didn't you say earlier it helps you relax and forget the pressure from your job?

CLIENT: Yes, that's right. I guess it helps me in my job by helping me keep my temper under control. The only other thing I can think of is it helps me meet people occasionally.

THERAPIST: Great. That certainly is a positive benefit. I imagine most of these people would be into staying fit?

CLIENT: That's true. Most avid cyclists are into being healthy. I'm not sure why I don't think about that more when I drink.

THERAPIST: That's an important question you're raising. Let's make sure we get back to it. Now, can you think of any financial benefits?

CLIENT: I had to invest some money into equipment initially, but on a daily basis it's cheaper than drinking.

THERAPIST: Let me just raise one possible legal benefit. There's no chance that you would get stopped for a DWI on your way home from the Exchange if you went cycling instead in the first place.

CLIENT: True!

It is important for the therapist to spend time probing this topic so that there is no question about what the client finds reinforcing. Behaviors or activities that are reinforcing in many different areas of the client's life probably will be good candidates for behaviors that can compete with drinking.

♦ ♦

This chapter has presented CRA's initial assessment protocol. The rationale for each component and instructions regarding implementation have been outlined. In reading the remainder of the text it will become apparent that these tools are utilized regularly throughout treatment. Sometimes they simply serve as reference points or reminders about reinforcers, while at other times they can be readministered to monitor progress and update treatment plans. As with many therapies, CRA's assessment and treatment processes are intentionally intertwined.

Appendix 2.A CRA FUNCTIONAL ANALYSIS FOR DRINKING BEHAVIOR (INITIAL ASSESSMENT)

Triggers		Behavior	Short-Term Positive Consequences	Long-Term Negative Consequences
External	Internal			
1. Who are you usually with when you drink?	1. What are you usually thinking about right before you drink?	1. What do you usually drink?	1. What do you like about drinking with _____ ? (who)	1. What are the negative results of your drinking in each of these areas: a) Interpersonal:
2. Where do you usually drink?	2. What are you usually feeling physically right before you drink?	2. How much do you usually drink?	2. What do you like about drinking _____ ? (where)	b) Physical:
			3. What do you like about drinking _____ ? (when)	c) Emotional:

34

3. When do you usually drink?

3. What are you usually feeling emotionally right before you drink?

3. Over how long a period of time do you usually drink?

4. What are some of the pleasant thoughts you have while you are drinking?

5. What are some of the pleasant physical feelings you have while you are drinking?

6.. What are some of the pleasant emotional feelings you have while you are drinking?

d) Legal:

e) Job:

f) Financial:

g) Other:

Appendix 2.B   CRA FUNCTIONAL ANALYSIS FOR DRINKING BEHAVIOR (INITIAL ASSESSMENT)

Triggers		Behavior	Short-Term Positive Consequences	Long-Term Negative Consequences
External	**Internal**			
1. <u>Who</u> are you usually with when you drink? *Fred and Bill*	1. What are you usually <u>thinking</u> about right before you drink? *I can't stand my boss. He doesn't treat me fair.*	1. <u>What</u> do you usually drink? *Miller beer*	1. What do you like about drinking with <u>*Fred & Bill*</u>? (who) *They hate the boss too. We all make fun of him.*	1. What are the negative results of your drinking in each of these areas: a) Interpersonal: *Gloria gets mad when I miss dinner.* *Got into an argument at the bar.*
			2. What do you like about drinking at the <u>*Exchange*</u>? (where) *It's close to work*	b) Physical: *Got a glass smashed on my hand. Had to get stitches.*
2. <u>Where</u> do you usually drink? *the Exchange*	2. What are you usually <u>feeling</u> physically right before you drink? *shaky*	2. <u>How much</u> do you usually drink? *5–6 12 oz bottles*	3. What do you like about drinking <u>*after work*</u>? (when) *It's a good time to unwind*	c) Emotional: *I get upset when Gloria is upset with me for getting home late.*

36

3. When do you usually drink?	3. What are you usually feeling <u>emotionally</u> right before you drink?	3. Over <u>how long</u> a period of time do you usually drink?	4. What are some of the pleasant <u>thoughts</u> you have while you are drinking?	d) Legal:
after work (3 weeknights)	mad inadequate embarrassed	approx. 2 hrs.	I'm not a bad guy. The boss is just a jerk	2 DWI's
			5. What are some of the pleasant <u>physical feelings</u> you have while you are drinking? I enjoy the taste of the beer. It's relaxing.	e) Job: Missed work when I got stitches
			6. What are some of the pleasant <u>emotional feelings</u> you have while you are drinking? less worrying. it's relaxing.	f) Financial: Health insurance didn't cover the stitches. Gloria will lose her wages for that time. g) Other:

Appendix 2.C CRA FUNCTIONAL ANALYSIS FOR <u>NONDRINKING BEHAVIOR</u> (_____)
(behavior/activity)

Triggers		Behavior	Short-Term Negative Consequences	Long-Term Positive Consequences
External	Internal			

External

1. <u>Who</u> are you usually with when you _____?
   (behavior/activity)

2. <u>Where</u> do you usually _____?

Internal

1. What are you usually <u>thinking</u> about right before you _____?
   (behavior/activity)

2. What are you usually <u>feeling physically</u> right before you _____?

Behavior

1. <u>What</u> is the nondrinking behavior/activity?

2. How <u>often</u> do you usually _____?

Short-Term Negative Consequences

1. What do you dislike about _____ with _____?
   (behavior/activity)   (who)

1. What do you dislike about _____?
   (behavior /activity)   (where)

1. What do you dislike about _____?
   (behavior /activity)   (when)

Long-Term Positive Consequences

1. What are the positive results of _____
   (behavior/activity)
   in each of these areas:
   a) Interpersonal:

   b) Physical:

   c) Emotional:

38

3. When do you usually
_____?

3. What are you usually feeling emotionally right before you _____?

3. How long does _____ usually last?

4. What are some of the unpleasant thoughts you usually have while you are _____?

d) Legal:

5. What are some of the unpleasant physical feelings you usually have while you are _____?

e) Job:

6.. What are some of the unpleasant emotional feelings you usually have while you are _____?

f) Financial:

g) Other:

39

Appendix 2.D CRA FUNCTIONAL ANALYSIS FOR NONDRINKING BEHAVIOR (_bike riding—weekday_)
(behavior/activity)

Triggers		Behavior	Short-Term Negative Consequences	Long-Term Positive Consequences
External	**Internal**			
1. Who are you usually with when you _ride_ ? (behavior/activity) *nobody*	1. What are you usually thinking about right before you _ride_ ? (behavior/activity) *looking forward to it helping me relax*	1. What is the nondrinking behavior/activity? *riding*	1. What do you dislike about _riding_ with _alone_ ? (behavior/activity) (who) *focus on aches & pains more*	1. What are the positive results of _riding_ (behavior/activity) in each of these areas: a) Interpersonal: *Relationship with Gloria is smoother.* *Helps me meet people occasionally*
2. Where do you usually _ride_ ? *near my home (on the main road)*	2. What are you usually feeling physically right before you _ride_ ? *less tense* *calmer*	2. How often do you usually _ride_ ? *2 weekday afternoons*	2. What do you dislike about _riding_ _on the main road_ ? (behavior/activity) (where) *feel like I'm going to get run off the road* 3. What do you dislike about _riding_ _after work_ ? (behavior/activity) (when) *traffic is heavy gets dark (so I have to hurry)*	b) Physical: *Keeps weight down.* *Good for blood pressure.* c) Emotional: *Reduces stress, so I feel better.* *Helps me relax & forget job pressure.*

3. When do you usually _ride_ ?

right after work
if I head straight
home on time —
I see other cyclists

3. What are you usually feeling emotionally right before you _ride_ ?

excited
happy

3. How long does _riding_ usually last?

an hour

4. What are some of the unpleasant thoughts you usually have while you are _riding_ ?

I better hurry or I'll
be late

5. What are some of the unpleasant physical feelings you usually have while you are _riding_ ?

get sore
feel tired

6.. What are some of the unpleasant emotional feelings you usually have while you are _riding_ ?

get mad at the drivers

d) Legal:
No chance of getting a
DWI.

e) Job:

helps keep my temper
under control

f) Financial:
it's cheaper than
drinking

g) Other:

41

3

Sobriety Sampling

Sobriety Sampling is a procedure that sets CRA apart from most other alcohol programs. It operates on the assumption that one can more successfully hook a client into treatment by not overwhelming him or her with rigid rules and frightening expectations. Specifically, Sobriety Sampling motivates the client to commit to stay abstinent for an agreed-upon, limited period of time. It is used with all clients, regardless of whether their final treatment goal is abstinence or moderation.

One must conceptually understand Sobriety Sampling to make the process work well. Most traditional alcohol programs in the United States use abstinence as their only drinking goal. In other words, clients are told that they *never* can drink again. The idea of staying abstinent for the rest of one's life is a concept that many people have great difficulty accepting, especially individuals who remain unconvinced that they have a drinking problem in the first place. Sobriety sampling plays an important role here. While it may be necessary ultimately for some clients to stay sober for the rest of their lives, Sobriety Sampling approaches this goal gently. It allows clients time to get accustomed to the idea that they may have a problem with drinking.

Advantages of a Sampling Approach

The Sobriety Sampling procedure serves many other useful purposes as well:

1. It allows you the opportunity to build rapport with a client while helping him or her recognize the severity of the problem.

2. It enables you and the client to set a goal together that the client feels is reasonable, appropriate, and obtainable. It does not frighten the client into deeper resistance.

3. It paves the way for the introduction of disulfiram (Antabuse) (See Chapter 4).

The remaining advantages of a sampling approach listed below may even be presented to a client to enhance motivation:

4. Having a "time-out" from drinking allows the client to experience the sensation of being sober. Typically this focuses attention automatically on positive changes in cognitive, emotional, and physical symptoms.

5. Sobriety Sampling actively disrupts old habits and drinking patterns, giving the client the opportunity to replace these behaviors with new positive coping skills.

6. Through setting and reaching attainable goals of short-term sobriety, clients learn self-reliance and control.

7. Realizing one's short-term goals serves as an experience of immediate and repeated success that then acts as a significant self-confidence enhancer and motivator.

8. Sobriety Sampling demonstrates the client's commitment to change, which in turn elicits the trust and support of family members.

9. This demonstrated commitment also slowly earns the confidence of law enforcement agencies (e.g., probation), which may have had negative encounters with the client due to his or her drinking.

10. Difficulty or relapse within a monitored sampling period can be used to illustrate where additional help is needed.

Introducing Sobriety Sampling

Sobriety Sampling consists of two phases: getting the client to agree to sample time-limited sobriety, and outlining a strategy for accomplishing this. The procedure used for the first phase, obtaining the commitment, is as follows:

1. Make sure you have reviewed the assessment material so that you know whether the client has had any recent periods of sobriety. In the

event that the person has, determine the typical length of the abstinent periods. This information may be useful later in the negotiating process if the client is reluctant to agree to a reasonable sampling period.

2. Also be sure you have noted in the assessment data the client's motivators for treatment. This information may be introduced as an incentive during the bargaining process.

3. Suggest that the client sample a time-limited period of sobriety. Mention several of the relevant sampling approach advantages just listed.

4. Next suggest that the sampling period be set for 90 days. Explain how the benefits derived from a sampling period appear to be best realized within such a time frame. Furthermore, you might also mention that since the first 90 days appears to be a high-risk relapse period (Marlatt, 1980), getting a firm commitment for 90 days of sobriety would be an excellent start.

5. If the client is unwilling to agree to 90 days, bargain downward. Your goal is to settle upon a time that appears to be a challenge, but one which is obtainable.

6. As noted above, be prepared to motivate the client by referring to previous periods of abstinence, or by reviewing the reasons for seeking treatment right now.

In the case example that follows, assume a client with a moderate but chronic alcohol problem appears for treatment for the first time. He is accompanied by his wife.

THERAPIST: Based on your assessment information and your functional analysis, it appears that you have had a difficult time trying to stay sober. Would that be a correct statement?

CLIENT: Yes, I have been drinking too much lately.

THERAPIST: And you've also stated, Ron, that this was pointed out to you by your son recently. Apparently he said that he wouldn't bring his family over for Sunday dinner anymore if you were going to drink and carry on like you have been. That must have had a big impact on you.

CLIENT: It did. It sort of shocked me. Personally, I think he exaggerated the whole thing.

THERAPIST: Maybe so. But what's important for us is that you're here, and that you've decided to do something about your drinking. Now, it also appears that you have not had any real extended period of sobriety. What would you like me to help you with?

CLIENT: I'm not sure. Maybe I should try to stay sober for awhile.

Note: The therapist relied on the assessment material to determine the client's typical length of recent abstinence and his motivation for treatment right now. This information may be used later to encourage a commitment to a reasonable period of sobriety. In this case the client alluded to a sampling period himself, so the therapist will support this idea by listing some of the pertinent benefits. Then he will suggest the relatively standard 90-day trial.

THERAPIST: It appears that you are truly motivated to make some changes in your life, and to take control of your actions. I agree with you; this would be a good time to see what it's like to be sober for a while. It's a great opportunity to try out new coping strategies, and to experience changes in thoughts and feelings just by being sober. And, of course, there's the issue of feeling more confident once you see yourself being successful. I bet your wife would really appreciate seeing you take a time-out from drinking, too. So a period of abstinence makes a lot of sense. And considering how determined you seem to be right now, I believe you would have no trouble at all staying sober for a minimum of 90 days.

CLIENT: Well, I don't know. That's a longer commitment than I was talking about. I don't think so.

THERAPIST: [Looking toward the wife]: Kathy, what do you think? Don't you think that Ron could stay sober for at least 90 days if he really wanted to?

WIFE: I feel that the decision is up to Ron, but I would love to see him sober that long.

THERAPIST: What do you think, Ron? Let's give it a try. Ninety days is nothing compared to a lifetime. All those benefits of sampling sobriety seem to come through loud and clear during a 90-day period of abstinence. Plus, you're at a greater risk for relapse during that time, so I'd be most comfortable with a 90-day commitment. What do you think?

Note: It was clear to the therapist from the assessment information that this client had had no extended period of sobriety, and consequently probably was not going to agree to a 90-day goal. Nevertheless, the therapist pushed for this at the start, linking the benefits of a sampling approach to a 90-day period. His main objective was to be certain that there would be ample room to bargain downward.

CLIENT: I just don't think that I want a goal of 90 days. Forget it.

THERAPIST: You seem to be really uncomfortable. I'm sorry if I've been too pushy. How would you feel about making a goal of 60 days? That would still give us a good opportunity to see some of those changes.

CLIENT: I just don't know. I'm not even sure that I have a real problem, or that I want to stay in this treatment program for 60 days.

THERAPIST: I bet you do have reservations about this process. It's totally new to you. I understand your hesitation. Why don't we just take it 30 days at a time? A month shouldn't be too difficult. And besides, the holidays are just a little bit more than a month away. Wouldn't it be nice to have 30 days of sobriety under your belt so that you could feel good about inviting your son and his family over for dinner?

CLIENT: I guess 30 days is OK.

THERAPIST: [*Looking to the wife*]: What do you think, Kathy?

CLIENT: I think it's great. Thirty days is a great start.

Note: The therapist tied in the 30-day goal with the client's main motivator: to maintain connections with his son and grandchildren. If this had been unsuccessful, the process would have continued until the client made any commitment, no matter how small. The therapist next would have asked for a 3-week commitment, then 2 weeks, and finally even just 1 day.

Planning for Time-Limited Sobriety

Once a decision has been made as to how long the client is going to remain sober, then the task at hand is to determine *how* exactly this will be accomplished. The important components of this second phase of Sobriety Sampling are:

1. Be sure to schedule the next appointment for a time that is no more than a few days away. Once a client is committed to attempting sobriety, it is essential to quickly teach skills necessary to be successful.

2. In devising a plan to stay sober, do not simply allow the client to rely on methods used in the past. Point out that these plans have not been very successful.

3. Have the client indicate which common drinking situation is the biggest threat to sobriety over the next few days. Refer to the client's functional analysis for that episode so that the main triggers can be reviewed. Check to see that the client still understands the concept of triggers, and remembers what they are.

4. Help the client develop a specific plan that relies upon alternative behaviors to compete with drinking during that high-risk occasion. Be sure that all of the triggers have been addressed.

5. Once a detailed plan has been worked out, instruct the client to develop a backup plan as well.

6. If necessary, remind the client of the motivators for making a best attempt at sobriety this time.

7. Reinforce the client whenever possible.

These points will be illustrated in the conversation that continues between Ron and his therapist:

THERAPIST: I'm real proud of your decision to sample sobriety for the next 30 days. That's a great goal. But since you have had problems in the past with sobriety, how will you accomplish your goal?

CLIENT: I guess I'll just not drink. If I use my willpower I think I can do it.

THERAPIST: I'm sure you can accomplish almost any reasonable goal you set for yourself, but, realistically speaking, you have not been very successful in the past trying to stay away from alcohol. Staying sober is not such an easy task. Has relying on your willpower ever kept you sober before?

CLIENT: Well, not for long. But this time I really mean it. I have to quit. I just can't keep going on the way I have been. Even my family's deserting me.

THERAPIST: I want to help you in every way that I can. Kathy, aren't you here, too, to help Ron in every way possible? Wouldn't you do everything in your power to promote his sobriety and well-being?

WIFE: Yes. I love Ron and I want to help in any and every way possible.

Note: Throughout this conversation the therapist turns to the wife when he feels certain that she will make a supportive, caring comment. Often this serves to further motivate the client.

THERAPIST: What are some other ways that you can meet your goal of 30 days of sobriety?

CLIENT: I'm not sure. I guess I could just go home right after work and stay there. I'll have to get rid of all the alcohol in my house so I'm not tempted.

THERAPIST: Has that technique ever worked in the past?

CLIENT: Not really. But I've never been in a program like this either.

THERAPIST: Ron, you've got a number of important things going for you this time. You've convinced me that you're motivated to change, and you know that if you do you'll be able to have your relatives over to the house again. And your wife has made it real clear that she's backing your efforts 100%. Also, you've got a good idea of where to start. You know that you need to go straight home after work, and get rid of all the alcohol in the house. I'd like to spend just a little more time figuring out what else we can set up so that you'll have the best chance of succeeding. Would you be willing to help me out with that?

CLIENT: I guess it wouldn't do any harm.

THERAPIST: OK. What we really need to do is to first schedule your next session for just a few days from now. I don't want to wait a whole week because there are some valuable skills that you need to learn in a hurry. So at your next session we'll go over basic problem-solving strategies. This will give you a specific procedure to follow when, for example, you get urges to drink.

CLIENT: Well, I hope it helps.

THERAPIST: I think it will, but we'll know for sure when you give it a try. So, will you be able to make your first problem-solving session this Friday at noon?

CLIENT: I don't see why not.

Note: It is necessary to proceed quickly with the various CRA techniques as soon as the client demonstrates some motivation to change. But it also is important not to overwhelm the client with too many procedures at once. Here the therapist first makes certain that the next session is scheduled for later that week, so that a strategy can be taught that will offer options for permanent change. In the meantime the therapist will pursue a simple temporary solution; namely, setting up behaviors that compete with drinking. He has made it clear to the client that it is insufficient to rely on past "strategies" to change his drinking behavior.

THERAPIST: Now, in the meantime, we should at least set up some behaviors that would compete with, or interfere with, your drinking. Ron, which of the common drinking situations that you included in your functional analysis would you say is the biggest obstacle to sobriety before we meet on Friday?

CLIENT: Probably just driving home from work each day and stopping at the corner convenience store on the way. I head straight home then with my beer and start in.

THERAPIST: Fine. Do you remember the triggers you listed for that type of drinking episode?

CLIENT: Some of them. As *soon* as I see the store and the beer advertisements in the window, the decision's already made. I start to think about how cold and satisfying that first beer is going to taste.

THERAPIST: OK Ron. You definitely had all of those triggers listed: the sight of the store and the beer advertisements in the window. Also, the thoughts about how it will taste going down. How about the *feelings* that are triggers?

CLIENT: Oh yeah. I always stop there on days that I'm feeling *really* tired.

THERAPIST: That's right. So now when you're heading home and you notice these triggers, you'll know that you need to act quickly or the drinking will win out. Which one do you notice first?

CLIENT: The tired feeling. I'm totally exhausted at least a couple of days each week. That starts me off.

THERAPIST: Let's find another way of dealing with the exhaustion. But first we need to get past the convenience store on the way home, since you just said that the decision to drink is already made once you see it.

CLIENT: Well, that's easy. I can just drive home a different route. There's lots of ways to get home from work.

Note: The therapist is reviewing the drinking triggers listed on the client's functional analysis. He checks to make sure both that the client still understands the concept of triggers, and that he remembers what his triggers are. The therapist proceeds with setting up alternative behaviors until all of the potential triggers have been addressed.

THERAPIST: OK. So you can go home an alternate route. But what happens if you're *real* tired? That's your first trigger to drink.

CLIENT: I guess I'll just ride it out.

THERAPIST: Maybe I can offer you something more than that. Ron, can you tell me *why* you drink beer when you get tired?

CLIENT: It wakes me up and makes me feel like doing something.

THERAPIST: What else could wake you up and make you feel alive? Do you drink coffee, or does a brisk walk wake you up?

CLIENT: I don't drink coffee and I've never liked walking. It's boring. But sometimes I go home and work in my yard. That keeps me going for awhile.

THERAPIST: Great. Can you commit to working in your yard each night after work, just until I see you again on Friday?

CLIENT: Sure. It's only a few days and there's a lot to do.

THERAPIST: How about a backup plan in the event of rain?

CLIENT: That's probably a good idea. I know, I could putter in the garage. I've been meaning to put up a shelf for a while.

THERAPIST: Fine. Let's summarize now. You're going to drive home a different way so you avoid the convenience store. And when you get home you'll work in the yard. If it's raining you'll put up a shelf in your garage.

CLIENT: Sure, I can do that.

THERAPIST: This will be a great start toward your goal to sample sobriety for 30 days.

As stated before, the therapist had two important tasks to accomplish: to get the client to agree to sample sobriety, and to outline with the client some specific strategy for staying sober. Clients frequently resist this second part, since they believe that it will be relatively easy to stay sober for just a few days. But you should stand firm about devising a concrete, new plan, because many clients will have difficulty trying to refrain from drinking even for a few days. Notice that the therapist also anticipated an obstacle: bad weather. Establishing even one backup plan introduces to the client the notion of planning for and dealing with obstacles. Remember, you want the client to experience success early in the program, so that motivation does not drop.

Selling Sobriety Sampling to a Resistant Client

Another example of the Sobriety Sampling procedure follows. The client in this scenario is more resistant to treatment and has a severe drinking problem. He was referred to the program through the court system. Regardless, the same two general components of Sobriety Sampling are covered: encouraging the client to commit to a sampling period, and devising a plan for achieving sobriety. The first category is illustrated in the segment of dialogue that follows.

Note that in presenting the advantages of a sampling period, you should only refer to those items which you believe will serve as motivators for your client. There is no reason to go down a long list of "advantages" if it is clear that the client will not view them as relevant. Also note that during the negotiation process for a sampling period with this difficult client, the therapist continually refers to the client's motivators. In this way arguments about the extent of the drinking "problem" are minimized, and an appeal for change is made to the client on a level which makes sense to him.

THERAPIST: Hi Dave. How are you doing today?

CLIENT: Not bad. How about you?

THERAPIST: Pretty good. Let's begin by talking about why you're here and how I can help you.

CLIENT: Well, I'm here because I got my third DWI, and if I don't come, I'll go to jail.

THERAPIST: Given the fact that you have three DWIs, it seems clear that your drinking has caused you considerable legal problems. Your assessment shows that drinking has created difficulties in other areas of your life also.

CLIENT: I don't drink as much as I used to. And most of my problems are due to bad luck, not drinking.

THERAPIST: Well, Dave, lots of people drink, but not all of them end up with three DWIs and a possible jail term. There may be more to your predicament than bad luck.

CLIENT: Well, I'm here, aren't I? So what do I have to do?

THERAPIST: You don't have to do anything if you don't want to. I'm just here to help if I can. Let me ask you a simple question. Do you think your drinking is a problem?

CLIENT: Not really.

THERAPIST: Do you think the judicial system thinks you have a problem with drinking and driving?

CLIENT: Big time. I almost went to jail.

THERAPIST: So at least in terms of the legal system, your drinking is a problem.

CLIENT: Yes, I guess so.

Note: The therapist did not spend time and energy arguing with the client over whether he had a drinking problem. Instead, she noted that the client's motivation for treatment was to avoid a jail sentence, and so she appealed to him logically in the legal arena. It appeared relatively easy for the client to accept such a label for his drinking behavior in that context. At this stage in the process, this was all the encouragement the therapist needed to introduce the notion of a period of sobriety.

THERAPIST: What shall we do about it? Do you want to quit for a while?

CLIENT: Supposedly it's part of my probation, but I'm still drinking. They don't know. You won't tell them, will you?

THERAPIST: Our sessions are confidential. But I must tell you, Dave, I'm here to help people stop abusing alcohol, not cheat the system. It looks like you do have a problem with alcohol, so my best advice is to stop drinking; at least for a short period of time so we can get a better look at things.

CLIENT: What's a short period?

THERAPIST: We can decide on that together. But first let me give you a few reasons why it's usually helpful to be abstinent for a while, even if abstinence isn't your ultimate goal.

CLIENT: This ought to be good.

THERAPIST: In your case it will demonstrate to your family and to the courts that you're serious about making some changes. The court system tends to look very favorably upon abstinence in situations like yours.

Note: The therapist presented only those "Advantages of a Sampling Approach" (p. 43) which she believed would be important to this particular client.

CLIENT: I know. I've thought about that. So like I said, what do you mean by a "short period"?

THERAPIST: How's 90 days sound? Ninety days of sobriety beats 90 days in jail.

CLIENT: No way! I didn't come here to quit. I don't really have a problem.

THERAPIST: Well, maybe not, but I always suggest to all my clients that they stop for 90 days. Some people find out that things actually get better in a lot of ways when they stop drinking. And if they don't, you can always start drinking again. But 90 days is considered a critical period, since most relapses happen during the first 3 months. Besides, don't you think it would take about 90 days of sobriety to really convince your family and the legal system that you were serious this time?

CLIENT: I'm not going to stop for 90 days. I don't drink that much anyway.

Note: The therapist again suggested a relatively long period of sobriety first, and gave a rationale for that choice. She knew in advance that bargaining would be a certainty.

THERAPIST: Well, if you don't drink that much, it should be easy to stop for a while. How about trying to quit for 60 days?

CLIENT: That's still too long. I don't want to make any deal to stop at all. Like I told you, I don't have a problem.

THERAPIST: That may be true, but the court system certainly sees it another way. And I think it might be a good challenge for you to see if you can quit even for a month, just to prove to yourself that you don't have a problem.

CLIENT: What do you mean, "to prove I don't have a problem"? I don't. I could quit if I wanted to. I just don't want to.

THERAPIST: Well, why don't you quit drinking for 2 weeks, and then we can talk in here about your experience of not drinking. Then I could write a favorable report to your probation officer. Just 2 weeks. Anybody can stay sober for 2 weeks, don't you think?

CLIENT: OK. I'll do it just to show you I can. I know you don't think I can stop for 2 weeks, but I can.

THERAPIST: Who knows, you may actually feel better physically and emotionally if you stop. It certainly can't hurt you.

Even in cases when you know the client should remain abstinent, Sobriety Sampling is used. Bonding with the client as opposed to alienating the individual is essential. This therapist also relied on two motivators to support her effort to get the client to sample sobriety for 2 weeks: (1) the therapist knew the client really believed he could stop if he wanted to, and that he would want to prove it to her, and (2) the client was told that a more favorable report to the probation officer could be written if he tried sobriety for 2 weeks. Use the motivators provided by the client to move the person in the desired direction.

Avoiding Confrontation While Establishing a Plan

It would be easy to become involved in a power struggle with this difficult client. This would accomplish nothing. Instead the therapist will avoid direct confrontation and still establish a specific, reasonable plan for achieving short-term sobriety. Refer to the section Planning for Time-Limited Sobriety (pps. 46–47) in this chapter for a listing of the steps.

THERAPIST: I usually like to see new clients twice each week for the first 2 weeks. Can you do that?

CLIENT: No way. I'm taking off work to be here. I can't afford any more time off.

THERAPIST: So I won't see you until next week. And I want to help you attain your goal of 2 weeks of sobriety. Let's look at the next week and see how we can improve your chances of making your goal.

Note: The therapist tried unsuccessfully to convince the client to attend twice-weekly sessions. She did not push the issue though, because it only would have resulted in a power struggle this early in treatment. For this same reason she will not make an issue out of his past unsuccessful, vague methods for curbing his drinking. Instead, she simply will present herself as an ally for achieving his goal.

CLIENT: If I say I'm going to stop, I'll do it!

THERAPIST: I'm on your side. I know you can do it. I just want to assist you. Can you help me out by telling me a situation that's likely to happen this week that will put you at the greatest risk for drinking?

CLIENT: If my girlfriend is late to pick me up from work. Sometimes I wait for 30 minutes and get so mad I leave and go to a bar. God, I hate it when she's late!

THERAPIST: And if I remember correctly we already filled out a functional analysis chart for that drinking episode.

CLIENT: We're not going to do that again, are we?

THERAPIST: I don't think we'll need to. I just want to make sure you remember your triggers for drinking in that situation.

CLIENT: It's pretty simple. I lose my temper. I usually go drink when I lose my temper.

THERAPIST: You're right; you had anger listed as a trigger. Do you remember any of your thoughts from that episode with your girlfriend?

CLIENT: Yes. I think things like, "I can't believe she's late again! I'd better get a beer to calm down."

THERAPIST: So you physically feel upset, too?

CLIENT: Definitely. Sometimes I can't sit still and my hands are shaking.

THERAPIST: You have a good memory. I won't go through the last few triggers, because they seem real clear to you. So your girlfriend picks you up after work every day. Sometimes she's late, and so you leave before she arrives and go drinking. How else could you handle this problem? What could you do instead of going to a bar and drinking?

Note: The therapist introduces the idea of an alternative behavior. It is extremely important that she do this, since this client is not going to be attending his first problem-solving session for an entire week.

CLIENT: I wouldn't have to rely on her for a ride in the first place if I could just get my driver's license back.

THERAPIST: That's true. And the best way to do that is to stay sober and show the legal system that you're a responsible citizen. But that's a long-term goal. How about a more immediate solution?

CLIENT: I know a guy who lives pretty close to my house. Maybe I could give him some gas money and he could drive me home for a week.

THERAPIST: That sounds like an excellent solution. For now it's even better than figuring out a new way to deal with your anger toward your girlfriend. We can do that later. This way you won't even have an opportunity to get upset in the first place. Do you think this guy will go for it?

CLIENT: Yes, he's always complaining about money, so if I give him some cash I know he'll do it.

THERAPIST: Is there a chance that this guy will be late someday, and you'll end up getting angry and drinking?

CLIENT: Not really. He gets off work the same time I do. He always goes straight home, as far as I know.

THERAPIST: Let's have a simple backup plan just in case. Suppose for some reason he's not quite ready to leave when you are. Make believe you feel yourself getting angry. What could you do besides drink to calm yourself down?

CLIENT: Hmmm. There's an employee lounge I could check out. I think there's a TV in it. I guess I could smoke a cigarette there and wait.

THERAPIST: Sounds like a good plan.

Note: Here the therapist not only encouraged the client to develop a backup plan, but she directly addressed the anger trigger. Planning to avoid the potential for an angry response to his girlfriend seemed reasonable in this case as a temporary solution. But an even better tactic was to have a strategy worked out in the event that he did become angry.

THERAPIST: OK, let's try this plan for the next week. Then we'll continue with actual problem-solving training, so that you'll learn a better way to handle your anger in the future without drinking.

The therapist deflected the aggressive style of the client on several occasions by moving forward with the business at hand: to decrease the likelihood that he would drink before their next session. By avoiding direct confrontation she was able to work with the client to find a suitable plan for the upcoming week. One should note carefully that the therapist was not coaxing the client to say that he would stay sober the rest of his life. Doing so would have resulted in the client terminating prematurely, or setting a goal that he had no intention of working toward. The client definitely did not appear ready to stop drinking for any extended period of time.

♦ ♦

Too often clients will not return to therapy if they receive the message that they can never drink again. Treatment programs lose their effectiveness quickly if clients drop out. CRA's Sobriety Sampling procedure safeguards against this outcome. It guides the client in a positive direction by avoiding confrontation as much as possible, and by relying on reinforcement and support. It approaches abstinence in a gentle, reasonable manner by trying to thread together sobriety even in small amounts. The "one day at a time" principle applies here. The next chapter introduces another tool, disulfiram (Antabuse), that can be incorporated into the second phase of the Sobriety Sampling procedure.

4

Disulfiram Use Within CRA

CRA teaches clients to utilize resources in their environment to promote a healthy lifestyle. For some this means adding disulfiram (Antabuse) to their treatment plan. Disulfiram is a medication that acts to deter the use of alcohol. Taken as prescribed, it is rare to experience any side effects unless alcohol is ingested. However, a disulfiram-ethanol reaction occurs if alcohol is imbibed while the client is using disulfiram. This chemical reaction causes the client to become extremely ill and prevents him or her from feeling the pleasurable effects of alcohol. This medication is particularly useful for those clients who repeatedly fail in their attempts to stop drinking, who face very serious consequences for continued drinking, who are prone to drink impulsively, and who have numerous drinking triggers. Disulfiram is an optional part of CRA treatment that can be beneficial in the recovery process for some clients. As noted in Chapter 1, disulfiram was later added to CRA's Sobriety Sampling procedure to assist in establishing a period of abstinence.

Recognizing the Need for Disulfiram as a Treatment Component

The conversation that follows is between a CRA therapist and a client with a severe alcohol problem. The medical, marital, and employment difficulties created by his drinking have prompted him to seek treatment. Assume that the therapist already has introduced the idea of Sobriety Sampling, and the client has made a commitment for 30 days. The dialogue begins with the therapist inquiring about Alberto's strategy for accomplishing this. Note the application of the steps listed under Planning for Time-Limited Sobriety (Chapter 3, pp. 46–47).

THERAPIST: Alberto, I'll do everything I can to help you achieve those 30 days of sobriety. Now, you said that in the past the only way you were able to keep from drinking for even 10 days was by being in the hospital. So if I ask you how in the world you are going to stay sober for 30 days when you're at work, at home, out in the community, and not locked up in a hospital, what would you say? How are you going to stay sober?

CLIENT: I guess I just won't drink.

THERAPIST: OK. But I bet you could use some help with that. Let's plan to meet again real soon so I can start teaching you some specific techniques.

CLIENT: Yes, sure. I can come this same time on Wednesday. Is that OK?

THERAPIST: That's fine. In the meantime let's identify what you see as the biggest challenge to sobriety over the next couple of days. Where are you most likely to be tempted to drink?

CLIENT: I'm not sure I can name one place. I suppose after work is the worst, but sometimes I have something to get me started in the morning. And lately we've all been heading out for a few beers at lunchtime, too.

Note: The therapist arranges for another session, and then attempts to identify the client's greatest threat to sobriety. It becomes apparent that there are many high-risk situations and even more triggers.

THERAPIST: This isn't going to be easy, Alberto. It would really help to have a specific plan to follow this time. I want you to be successful, so we need to come up with a plan that goes beyond just willpower.

CLIENT: Well . . . I guess I could pour out all the booze that's in my house. And I guess I could drive myself to work and come home right after work.

THERAPIST: Have you ever told yourself in the past, "I'm just going to go right home from work. I'm not going to have anything to drink?"

CLIENT: Thousands of times.

THERAPIST: And what happened?

CLIENT: Well, I get with the guys, it's right after work, it's hot outside . . . construction you know . . . .

THERAPIST: And you start drinking.

CLIENT: Yeah. And someone usually comes up and has a cooler in the truck and we stop by a bar and have a couple. We start having a good time and that's it. Once I start I just can't stop.

THERAPIST: What you're telling me then, is that you may have a plan, but you don't think it can work. And you're really not sure how you can stay sober for 30 days, but you're willing to give me a 30-day commitment to stop.

CLIENT: I have to. I want my family. My wife's going to kick me out, and I want to keep my job. And I don't want to die. My doctor says I'm digging my own grave by drinking the way I do.

The therapist makes it clear that, despite the client's good intentions, without a solid plan this time he will have very little chance of honoring his commitment to abstain. While attempting to establish this specific plan, it becomes apparent to the therapist that disulfiram could be an excellent addition to the treatment program. To begin with, this client is subjecting himself to many serious consequences if he continues to drink. Furthermore, he has made numerous unsuccessful attempts to control his alcohol consumption in the past. Finally, because he is drinking frequently and in so many different places, it would be impossible to address all the triggers and set up competing behaviors.

Presenting Disulfiram as an Effective Treatment Component

As the dialogue continues, the therapist will suggest that disulfiram be considered a viable treatment supplement. The basic facts that will be emphasized include:

1. Disulfiram is a powerful deterrent to drinking, because you will become very sick if you ingest alcohol while using it.
2. The deterrent effect lasts up to 2 weeks after you stop taking disulfiram.
3. There are many advantages to being on disulfiram (see Advantages of Disulfiram, pp. 62–64).
4. Disulfiram is only one part of the CRA program. Therapy sessions will continue to focus on other problems.
5. Disulfiram seems to work best as an adjunct to treatment if a trained monitor participates in the procedure. This person should attend the next session.

THERAPIST: Alberto, you have to work with me here. You want to stay sober for 30 days, and you've given me that commitment, even without a plan. What if I told you that there was something you could do, a special tool you could use that would help you stay sober for 30 days? Now, you're working construction. You know how important it is to have the right tool for the right job. I have a tool available for you. Would you be willing to consider using a tool to help you stay sober and reach your goal?

CLIENT: Like Valium?

THERAPIST: No, not like Valium. Valium wouldn't really help you reach your goal. It could actually do the opposite, because Valium is a drug, too, like alcohol. And I think it would be very detrimental if you got hooked on Valium and started using that in place of alcohol.

CLIENT: I guess you're right about that. Last time the doctor gave me Librium. I took that and drank on top of it. In fact, it made me feel like I wanted to drink.

THERAPIST: I wouldn't send you to get Librium. Now, back to staying sober for those 30 days. What if I told you that I had a tool in the form of a little white pill? Taken every day, this pill would help you stay sober because this pill would make it impossible for you to feel the "good effects" of alcohol. You would never get the "high" from the alcohol because it would make you sick.

CLIENT: Now come again. If I take this pill, I can drink all I want and not get drunk?

THERAPIST: No. If you take this pill and drink on top of it, it will make you very, very sick. It will make you throw up; it will make you dizzy, give you cold and hot sweats, shivers, and prickly heat.

CLIENT: Sounds bad.

THERAPIST: That's the idea. This is called a deterrent. And what we're trying to do is to deter you; to keep you from using alcohol. And since we haven't come up with a really concrete plan, I recommend that you use this drug, disulfiram. It definitely will help you stay away from alcohol, because if you drink while using it, you will become very, very sick.

CLIENT: So if I drank . . . anything at all?

THERAPIST: That's right.

CLIENT: Just like when I drink too much.

THERAPIST: Well, similar, but actually it could be worse than that.

CLIENT: Do I have to take this drug every day?

THERAPIST: You just have to take it for the 30 days you've made a commitment for.

CLIENT: Now, let's say that I take this drug, but within 3 days I have to have a drink. I can't make it. What happens?

THERAPIST: That's a very good question. The drug has what is called a residual effect; it stays in your bloodstream for about 7 to 14 days after you stop taking it. If you decide to drink; if you can't fight off those feelings, and you stop taking the disulfiram, you will still have it in your system for up to 2 weeks. This means you can't safely drink. There is still a chance that you'll become ill.

CLIENT: So I'd still have to stay sober for a while after stopping it?

THERAPIST: Yes, that's true. And you'd certainly have the right to quit the plan whenever you wanted to. But if you did decide to change our plan, I'd want you to call me first. Remember, we'd be meeting between one and two times each week throughout this 30-day period. So while we're working on your problems in other areas, you could tell me how the disulfiram is working out.

Note: The therapist explains how disulfiram acts as a deterrent to drinking, and adds that the residual effects can last for 2 weeks. She also makes it clear that disulfiram is only one part of the comprehensive treatment plan. The therapist then follows through with the Sobriety Sampling step of arranging a backup plan. In this case it would be to call her if the client decided to stop taking disulfiram.

CLIENT: I've never taken a drug like this. I don't know what it would be like to know I can't drink.

THERAPIST: I can certainly understand your apprehension. Let me tell you some of the benefits of taking disulfiram. Maybe that will make you feel like your efforts are worthwhile. First, you would have a more trusting relationship with your wife because she'd know you were taking it. Your boss would feel better about you because you'd be trying to do something very concrete. You wouldn't just be paying lip service; you'd actually be taking a drug that would help you stay away from alcohol so you could do a better job. It's also useful because it doesn't allow you to drink impulsively. Because of the residual effects, you'd have to decide several days in advance that you were going to drink. That alone would help you control your urges. Plus, it would help you stay in therapy so that you could work on your problems. And there are really minimal side effects from the drug if you don't drink while on it.

Note: The therapist reviews some of the benefits of taking disulfiram (see pp. 62–64 for a complete description of advantages).

THERAPIST: Do you have any questions, Alberto?

CLIENT: Not really. The whole thing sounds kind of scary.

THERAPIST: Well, so does dying from alcoholism too.

CLIENT: Well, I'll try it. For 30 days.

THERAPIST: Good. Now I'd like to have your wife come in so that she can be part of this. Disulfiram treatment works best when someone gives it to you and praises you for taking it. I'd like to have your wife be this person.

Note: A description of the actual disulfiram administration procedure will be presented in conjunction with an explanation of the duties of the disulfiram monitor.

Advantages of Disulfiram

Clients may offer various rationales for not taking disulfiram. One way to promote the use of the drug is to enumerate the many advantages of being on disulfiram:

1. *Reduction in Family Worry*: Taking disulfiram in the prescribed way decreases family worry about future drinking episodes. Discuss with the client whether the Concerned Other ever appears upset when the client leaves the house, even when there is no intention of drinking. Explain that the Concerned Other would be more relaxed and better able to relate in a positive way if the apprehension about the client potentially going out to drink could be reduced.

2. *Increase in Family Trust*: Taking disulfiram demonstrates to family members the client's commitment to stop drinking. This is an important step, because oftentimes the trust level is too low to even begin to work on relationship issues. Discuss with the client and the Concerned Other the number of times a verbal commitment was made and not kept. When a client is using disulfiram there is tangible evidence that he or she truly is working on attaining sobriety. Consistent with the CRA approach, it leaves nothing to chance.

3. *Reduction in "Slips"*: When a client is taking disulfiram it decreases the chance of experiencing demoralizing "slips" that could otherwise impede counseling progress. Also, a slip could elicit the Abstinence Violation Effect (Marlatt & Gordon, 1985) and have devastating consequences. The Abstinence Violation Effect occurs when clients have one drink and then rationalize that they might as well continue drinking, since they "blew it" already anyway. A related issue is the fact that some clients do not believe they have the ability to control their drinking once they have started. Therefore, potential slips should be actively avoided.

4. *Increase in Ability to Address Many Drinking Triggers at Once*: Before a client has had the opportunity to learn the basic CRA techniques, most therapists simply help the individual set up alternative behaviors that interfere with drinking. But this is extremely difficult to do if a client reports a wide variety of drinking episodes and innumerable triggers. Taking disulfiram is one way to simultaneously address every temptation to drink.

5. *Increase in Productive Therapy Time*: A client on disulfiram has time to deal constructively with current life problems, such as anxiety, other drug use, marital problems, and unemployment. This client can look objectively at his or her drinking patterns and address stressful antecedents. Total sobriety is the best condition under which good decisions can be made about one's life.

6. *Increase in Reliance Upon Other Coping Skills*: As noted, disulfiram prevents impulsive drinking through its residual effects. So assume that a client is accustomed to relieving anxious and agitated feelings by drinking alcohol. This is no longer a viable coping strategy if a person is taking disulfiram. Instead, the client is forced to develop alternative tactics to handle stress.

7. *Increase in Self-Confidence*: Since a client using disulfiram cannot drink spontaneously, the individual will have the opportunity to experience how cravings typically dissipate without resorting to alcohol. This "victory" will empower the client—the individual will gain confidence in the ability to control or reduce personal problems. As a result, alcohol will lose some of its importance.

8. *Reduction in Complicated, Agonizing Daily Decisions*: Disulfiram makes the decision process regarding whether to stay sober much simpler, because the client has only one decision to make each day: whether or not to take the pill. Most clients can relate to this, for they wrestle several times daily with the question of whether or not they should drink, or how much they should drink. The mental gymnastics clients experience often drain them of much of their energy and weaken them to the point where they drink just to end the debate!

9. *Increase in Opportunities for Positive Reinforcement*: When disulfiram is taken according to the specified procedure with a monitor, it provides the client with a daily reminder of his or her commitment to change, and an opportunity to be praised by the Concerned Other who is administering the medication.

10. *Increase in Available Early Warning Signs*: When a client is using disulfiram it provides the monitor with a concrete Early Warning System regarding the client's intention to drink. This Early Warning System (see Chapter 10: CRA Relapse Prevention) is a procedure in which the Concerned Other is trained to be sensitive to the antecedents of the client's drinking behavior. The client's refusal to take

disulfiram is one of the most obvious signs of an impending relapse. Interventions to prevent relapse at such threatening times are taught and rehearsed.

Involving the Client's Family Physician

Disulfiram use should be initiated by having the client sign a specific consent form that acknowledges a clear understanding of the dangers of drinking alcohol while on disulfiram (see Appendix 4.A). Next, a physician who is familiar with disulfiram will need to be contacted so that he or she may examine the client, and if appropriate, prescribe and medically monitor the disulfiram. The physician will be looking for a number of potential contraindications for disulfiram use, including liver disease, heart disease, a history of psychosis, and pregnancy.

Involving a physician in the care of a client will require a signed release form from the client, even if the individual is the client's family doctor. In many instances it will be worthwhile to send a letter to this physician, indicating that the ramifications and effects of the disulfiram have been discussed with the client. (Some CRA therapists enclose a copy of the signed Disulfiram Consent form as well.) Furthermore, this letter should state that disulfiram will only be part of the entire treatment program (see Appendix 4.B). But despite your efforts to educate and document, occasionally problems arise when a family physician refuses to cooperate. Often this individual is relatively unfamiliar with alcohol treatment or disulfiram. Having an alternative physician available is then desirable.

Refusal of Disulfiram

Even the most highly respected and well-trained therapists occasionally are faced with good disulfiram candidates who absolutely refuse to take the drug. The dialogue that follows shows a therapist conducting the second phase of Sobriety Sampling: Planning for Time-Limited Sobriety (see Chapter 3, pp. 46–47). Although it becomes apparent that the client is a solid candidate for disulfiram use, he is adamant about being able to achieve sobriety without it. He maintains this attitude despite hearing about the advantages of disulfiram. Since the therapist was taught to adhere to the CRA philosophy of "take what is given", he refrains from entering into a power struggle. He does suggest that the client sign a contract, however, in which he states his willingness to try disulfiram if, after a month, he has not been successful in abstaining without it.

THERAPIST: Great, Mike. That's the attitude. I'm glad you've agreed to abstain from drinking for 30 days. Now, before you leave today, let's set up another session for real soon. There are some things I can teach you that will make staying sober easier. But in the meantime, let's at least get an idea of what you think are going to be the most difficult times in terms of resisting alcohol this week.

CLIENT: Yeah . . . it might be a tough week to start this because I already know about a softball game and a company picnic. We always drink at those. And because it's been so hot, we've been going out for drinks most nights after work.

THERAPIST: Remember when we talked about triggers for drinking?

CLIENT: Yep. My friends are the biggest triggers. And we're together most of the time. We even work together.

THERAPIST: So what kind of plan do you have to make sure you don't drink? I imagine it's not realistic to think you can stay completely away from your main triggers.

Note: The therapist has mentioned scheduling another appointment soon, and has drawn attention to high-risk events and the relevant triggers. Due to the extent of the drinking and the number of unavoidable triggers, it would be very difficult to establish competing behaviors. The stage is being set for the introduction of disulfiram.

CLIENT: I just won't drink! When I say I'm going to quit, my word's pretty good. I'm known for my word.

THERAPIST: In the past, have you ever said, "I'm going to quit," and it just didn't happen that way?

CLIENT: Lots of times.

THERAPIST: Lots of times. So what makes this time different? How are you going to be able to stay sober this time when all those other times failed?

CLIENT: I guess I'll just have to cut it out. I'll just come home early from work. And maybe I'll tell the guys that the doctor told me I had to cut back. Like this is a test or something.

THERAPIST: You think that'll be successful, I mean, with the guys? Do you think they'll care what the doctor says?

CLIENT: Well, they're my friends. I hope so.

Note: The therapist impresses upon the client the low likelihood of success if he insists on trying to control his drinking the same ways he has in the past.

THERAPIST: I would hope so, too. But what if that doesn't work? What if I told you there was another way, using a tool—a tool to help you stay away from drinking?

CLIENT: Sounds good.

THERAPIST: Ever heard of a pill called Antabuse, which is a small...

CLIENT: Isn't that the pill that makes you sick and throw up?

THERAPIST: It would only make you sick if you drank while taking the pill.

CLIENT: Yep. There was a guy at work that was on it and he got real sick. Nah, I don't want anything to do with that.

THERAPIST: That means he drank then. See, I don't think . . .

CLIENT: No. I don't want to take it.

THERAPIST: But Mike, you seem too sensible of a guy to drink on disulfiram. And you said you really want to quit. So why don't you give it a try? Being on Antabuse would ensure that you wouldn't give in to impulsive urges to drink. It would make your wife feel better, because she wouldn't have to worry every day about whether or not you were going to drink. That alone would improve your relationship with her. And maybe your old boss would even take you back full-time if he knew you'd made a commitment and backed it up with medication. I've seen it happen before. In the meantime we could get a good start in therapy working on some of your other problems.

Note: The therapist reminds the client of his motivators to stay sober, informs him about some of the advantages of using disulfiram, and makes it clear that disulfiram is only part of the treatment.

CLIENT: Nah. I think I'd rather try on my own. I mean, what you're saying makes sense, but I think I can do it without any crutch this time.

THERAPIST: So, you're saying, then, that for 30 days, on your own, you're not going to drink any alcohol whatsoever.

CLIENT: I've said it.

THERAPIST: OK. I think it's really important that you take disulfiram. But I'm going to go with your decision—for up to a month.

CLIENT: So, you're going to let me try it on my own for 30 days?

THERAPIST: That's correct. Of course, we'll be meeting in a few days, so you can let me know how it's going then.

CLIENT: If I drink anything at all, then what?

THERAPIST: Then maybe we should try the disulfiram for 30 days. Just for 30 days. If you don't like it, or if there's a problem, you can stop. But 30 days of your life is nothing compared to how many days you've been drinking. It's a very short investment in your life.

CLIENT: OK. Well, let me do it my way. I still think I can quit on my own.

THERAPIST: How about we draw up a contract? I want to make sure we don't have any misunderstanding down the road. Is that OK with you?

CLIENT: You mean write down that I'm not going to drink for 30 days, and if I do I have to take that drug?

THERAPIST: That's basically correct. But remember, Mike, that you will be *choosing* to take disulfiram. You will not be forced at any time.

CLIENT: OK. I can live with that.

Note: Since the client absolutely refused to start on disulfiram, the therapist allowed him to attempt to stop drinking on his own for a limited period of time. But he had the client sign a contract whereby he agreed to take disulfiram if sobriety became impossible to attain. It is necessary, however, for the therapist still to assist the client in preparing a plan for achieving sobriety without the use of disulfiram.

THERAPIST: OK, Mike. Now let's come up with a simple strategy for how you're going to stay sober until our next appointment. At that time we can start working on a specific problem-solving technique that will help you regularly in the future. But for now, what are some things you'll need to do differently this week to increase your chances of success? Think of your high-risk drinking times and the triggers that we talked about earlier. And let's not forget a backup plan!

The therapist is now in a win–win situation. If the client stays sober, the therapist can work with this success. If the client resumes drinking, he can be shown how difficult it is to stay sober without "help." At that point the therapist would produce the contract to remind the client of his abstinence goal and the disulfiram option.

Concerned Other Support

Even though the client was unwilling to take disulfiram, it is still important to involve a Concerned Other in the treatment program as early as possible (see Chapter 9: CRA Marital Therapy). In this next scenario the therapist speaks to Mike's wife about her significant role in helping her husband achieve sobriety. He spends much of the time discussing disulfiram, as he believes it would be highly beneficial in Mike's case. The therapist presents an overview of how disulfiram works and its many advantages. During this process he is evaluating whether Mike's wife would be a good candidate for the disulfiram monitor. He is interested in her commitment to the relationship, and her ability to be supportive. Since she appears to be a suitable candidate, he later briefly describes how she would present the disulfiram. He also requests that she avoid broaching the topic with Mike, that she leave it up to the therapist.

THERAPIST: Marta, I wanted to talk with you today about your husband's drinking. Maybe you and I can do something together to try and help Mike deal with his problem. Would you like to discuss it?

WIFE: Yes.

THERAPIST: It's apparent that in the past Mike has had a severe problem with alcohol, and that it has caused you a lot of pain.

WIFE: Well, you know, I think Mike has always been an alcoholic. His father died of alcoholism. Mike's a wonderful father and he's good to the kids, but when he drinks he gets real moody. We fight. If he doesn't quit now, I'm leaving him. I can't take it anymore.

THERAPIST: It sounds like you've been through a lot of difficult times. There's a couple of different ways we can deal with this together. First, we'll need to get you active in the therapy with him. Part of the therapy could involve a special tool that will help him stay sober. As you know, Marta, people often stop drinking for short periods of time, but eventually start in again. They end up feeling guilty, and sometimes are more upset than they were before they quit. This can be very devastating. Have you seen this happen to Mike over the years?

WIFE: Oh yeah. I know he means well. I know he'd probably like to stop. He just can't do it.

THERAPIST: So it seems like he can't do it. But you are still willing to try and help? I know it's not your problem directly. But as long as you're with Mike and he's supporting the kids, obviously it's going to have an impact on the happiness in your lives. Do you really feel like you want to put some effort into this?

WIFE: I am willing to do pretty much anything.

Note: The therapist is forming an alliance with his client's wife, for he feels she could play a significant role in the therapy process. He also is evaluating whether she would be a good candidate for the disulfiram monitor. She appears to be committed to the marriage, and willing to help her husband stay sober.

THERAPIST: I want to describe to you a drug called disulfiram. Have you ever heard of disulfiram or Antabuse?

WIFE: No.

THERAPIST: Disulfiram, basically, is a little white pill, about the size of an aspirin. If your husband took this pill every day, he wouldn't be able to drink without getting very sick. The purpose of disulfiram is to deter him; to make him afraid of drinking even the smallest quantities. If he drank even one beer or a half of a beer, he could become very sick. Disulfiram would give your husband a chance to stay sober and in therapy long enough to work out some of the problems and difficulties that got him to this particular point in his life. It also would directly help your relationship by building some trust. Obviously, he's told you he's going to quit several times, and nothing long term ever came of it. Is that correct?

WIFE: Hundreds of times. I don't know if I can believe him. He says he's going to stay sober and never does.

Note: The therapist presents some of the advantages of disulfiram treatment (see pp. 62–64).

THERAPIST: Would you like to help him? Would you like to give him the best chance possible of staying sober?

WIFE: Like I said, I'd do anything. I love him when he's not drinking.

THERAPIST: I have asked him to stay sober for 30 days. He's going to try doing it his own way for those 30 days. If he's unsuccessful, he says he will then come back and try this drug called disulfiram.

WIFE: Do you really think he's going to stay sober?

THERAPIST: Well, I really don't know, but I am willing to let him try his way. But I did ask him to sign a contract to take disulfiram if he fails his way. We do that a lot. I like Mike and I want to help him, but there is no sense in banging heads. Now if he comes back and tells me he drank, I really need your help to become what we call a disulfiram monitor. I am not putting the responsibility for Mike's drinking on you; I'm only asking you to support Mike by helping him take disulfiram if it comes to that. We'll talk about how you would give it to him every day.

Note: The therapist makes it clear that the wife would have a very significant role as the monitor: to be supportive. At the same time, it would not be her job to feel guilty and responsible if her husband started drinking again.

WIFE: So, if Mike agrees to take this, you want me to give it to him every day. He won't drink if he does, because he'd get real sick?

THERAPIST: That's exactly right. Now I would ask you to administer the disulfiram in a specific way, and to say something really supportive of Mike while doing so. And I'd explain to Mike that he'd be expected to respond in a caring way. But don't worry about the details now. We would go over all the necessary steps if and when the time comes.

WIFE: It all sounds great. I hope he decides to take it.

THERAPIST: Me too. But we need to give him some space. And it's important, Marta, that you let me bring up the topic of disulfiram with him again if necessary. Just in case he gets angry, I want him to focus it at me. I don't want to put you in a situation that's difficult for you. So, in the meantime, I'm going to give you some literature on disulfiram that discusses its benefits. Take it home and study it. If and when the time comes, I'll call you both back for further training.

In this case the therapist determined easily that the spouse would be a suitable monitor, as she was supportive and wanted to stay with her husband. So he described some of the relevant advantages of disulfiram to her, and briefly presented the monitor's role. In doing so, it was essential that the therapist not place too much responsibility on the spouse for the client's recovery. Instead, he simply gave her some constructive ways to be involved in the treatment. And, finally, he cautioned her to refrain from pursuing the disulfiram option with her husband. The therapist preferred to deal with the client directly on the matter, rather than risk placing the wife in a potentially inflammatory position.

The example just presented involved an individual therapy session with just the client's spouse. Another therapist might have decided to conduct essentially the same session, but with the client attending as well. One justification for meeting with the spouse alone was the therapist's strong belief that the client was eventually going to take disulfiram, despite his initial refusal. With this in mind, the therapist wanted to enlist the spouse's support as a monitor immediately. But an extensive disulfiram discussion in the presence of this client probably would have been viewed as a lack of therapist support for the client's efforts to achieve abstinence his own way. This easily could have undermined the therapeutic relationship.

Reintroducing the Client's Disulfiram Contract

The next dialogue is between the therapist and both Mike and Marta. Mike started to drink on Day 4. When he called on Day 5, an appointment for the couple was scheduled immediately. Note the points covered at the start of the session:

1. The therapist reinforces the client for calling as soon as he started drinking again.
2. The therapist reminds the client about the disulfiram contract from the previous session.
3. The therapist reviews the client's motivators for changing his behaviors now.
4. The therapist reminds the client of several of the advantages to being on disulfiram.

THERAPIST: Well, Mike, I'm really pleased that you gave me a call as soon as you started drinking. That shows true motivation, and I'm real excited about that. It shows that you really want to take control of your life.

CLIENT: Well, things just didn't work out.

THERAPIST: OK. But you're here now and you brought Marta with you. Let's not dwell on the past. Let's decide, together, how we can make it more likely that you will succeed this time. Do you recall that the last time you were here you made a contract to take disulfiram if you resumed drinking?

Note: The therapist reinforces the client for calling as soon as he started drinking again. Next the therapist moves forward in a positive way by stating that they will work together to come up with a better strategy. He reminds the client of the disulfiram contract.

CLIENT: Disulfiram. That's the pill that makes you sick.

THERAPIST: If you drink. Correct. And I should let you know that when Marta came in a few days ago, I also explained disulfiram to her.

CLIENT: Oh. OK.

THERAPIST: Mike, you tried on your own and you made it about 5 days. That's a good start, but I know you can do better.

CLIENT: It just didn't work out.

THERAPIST: What do you think will happen if you keep drinking? What about your job? And do you think Marta is going to continue struggling with you forever?

Note: The therapist is reminding the client about the motivators for changing his behavior.

CLIENT: I know she's at the end of her rope. I don't think I have any other choice but to try the disulfiram. I've even met with my doctor already about it. Here's his prescription for it.

THERAPIST: I think you're making a good decision. I'd like to send you right down to our pharmacy so you can have your prescription filled and take your first dose before you leave today. I'd suggest starting with a 30-day period. We can use that time constructively. We've talked before about how a month of sobriety will give us time to work on some issues between you and Marta. And it will also be useful for your boss to hear about your decision.

The client appears to be willing and medically eligible to take disulfiram. The therapist presents a positive perspective by reminding the client about some of the advantages to being on disulfiram. Assume now that the couple leaves to have the prescription filled, and then returns to the session.

The Monitoring System

When a client agrees to take disulfiram, steps must be taken to ensure that the individual uses it as prescribed. As mentioned earlier, a critical component of disulfiram treatment is having a monitor (Azrin et al., 1982). The monitor can be any concerned person who is willing to spend time and energy to assist the client. Typically the monitor is a spouse, a fellow employee, a close friend, or a boss. At times, however, police and probation officers have been utilized. Both the client and the monitor must understand that this is not a punitive role but a supportive one. It will not be effective if the monitor is viewed only as a watchdog.

With this understanding in mind, the steps listed below are covered during the first disulfiram administration session. Assume that the client has been medically cleared in advance by a physician as a suitable disulfiram candidate.

1. If the couple does not bring their disulfiram pills to the session, they are sent to have the prescription filled.
2. The therapist impresses upon the monitor how important it is to be extremely supportive during the administration procedure.

3. The therapist tells the couple it is critical for them to follow the steps of the procedure exactly:
    (a) Examine the pill to be certain that it is disulfiram. Place one whole 250-mg disulfiram pill in the bottom of a clear glass. (Note that the dose may vary, depending on the individual. Also, it is common to administer a 500-mg dose daily during the first week.)
    (b) Pour in a small amount of water (approximately 2 inches), until the glass is almost half full.
    (c) Allow the pill to dissolve for about 1 minute. Crush the remainder with a spoon.
    (d) Stir the mixture slowly, making sure that all the disulfiram is dissolved.
    (e) Give the glass to the client and watch him or her drink the contents. If there is some stuck to the side of the glass, pour in more water, swish it around, and ask the client to finish it.
    (f) Praise the client for taking the disulfiram and for all that he or she has achieved since deciding to stop drinking.
4. The therapist models supportive comments for the couple to make to each other during the procedure.
5. The therapist asks the couple to role-play the administration procedure, and offers reinforcement and feedback.
6. The couple is asked to describe their feelings about the process.
7. The therapist instructs the monitor to actually administer the first dose of disulfiram in accordance with the procedures.
8. Additional feedback and reinforcement are offered.
9. A specific time is selected for the daily disulfiram administration. It should be a time that the couple typically spends together (e.g., breakfast or bedtime), and one that is convenient for both.
10. The couple is asked to bring the pills to subsequent sessions so that their technique can be observed.

THERAPIST: Did you get the disulfiram OK? Any problems?

WIFE: Everything was fine.

THERAPIST: I appreciate your enthusiasm. Can I see your prescription? I want to show you, Marta, what the disulfiram looks like. As you can see, the pill says Antabuse on it. So this is the pill that you will be administering to your husband every day.

Note: The therapist is training the monitor to scrutinize the pill to determine if, in fact, it really is disulfiram. This is easiest when the name of the drug is inscribed on the pill itself, as with Antabuse. Clients have been known to pour out the disulfiram pills and replace them with vitamins or other inert ingredients.

THERAPIST: Let's first go over the procedure on how to administer it, and then you can actually take one. If you have any questions along the way, just ask. We're going to do every step in a positive, supportive way. Nobody's playing cops or acting as a watchdog. You are doing this because you love and care about each other, and because this procedure has been proven to be extremely effective. I want you to take the disulfiram in a very specific way: the way that works!

Note: The couple should understand that the procedure is most effective if followed exactly as described.

THERAPIST: Mike, you agreed to have Marta act as your disulfiram monitor. Is that correct?

CLIENT: Yes. She's going to watch me take it.

THERAPIST: She is going to *support* your taking it. Can you understand the difference?

CLIENT: It sounds to me like you guys don't trust me to take it on my own.

THERAPIST: Actually, we've learned that if a spouse is involved, she can support you, and you can work on your relationship at the same time.

WIFE: But I don't think I *would* trust him to take it on his own.

THERAPIST: Well, I can appreciate that because of past history. But what I would like for you to do now is to put that away for a while. We can talk about that later. During the disulfiram administration procedure, Marta, it's extremely important for you to be very supportive, and to think about how Mike is trying something new that is very hard for him to do. If he takes this pill, he can't drink. He will become very sick if he drinks anything. So he's making a serious commitment. Right now I would like a serious commitment from you to try to support him in a positive way and not to talk about anything negative. We can talk about the negative things that have happened because of his drinking at another time. Does that make sense?

WIFE: Yeah.

Note: The therapist would work on the wife's distrust at a later point in therapy. It is very important for the disulfiram administration procedure to be conducted in a positive and supportive manner.

THERAPIST: I really appreciate your support. I know this is awkward, but it will pay off in the long run. OK, first, I'd like Mike to give you the disulfiram, so that you can look at it. Good. Now drop it into a small glass, and put about 2 inches of water into it. Let it set for a minute and watch it dissolve. Go ahead and crush any remaining pieces against the side of the glass with a spoon. Then stir slowly to make sure it's all dissolved. Now let's practice the conversation you'll have. I would like you to look directly at Mike, not at me, while you're making your response. Look at Mike and tell him how you feel. Say something like this: "Mike, I really appreciate that you are taking the disulfiram. I care about you and I'm glad that you are trying to stop drinking." Can you do that Marta? Why don't you look at him and try it.

WIFE: I can't say it just like you did. [Looking at her husband] Umm . . . Mike, you know, I'm really happy that you want to stay sober. I'm happy that you're taking this disulfiram and trying to work on our relationship.

THERAPIST: That was excellent. First of all, you looked at him. You were very positive, and you told him how you felt. You did a really good job. Now, Mike, just pretend that she's giving you the disulfiram. Make believe you are drinking it, and then practice thanking Marta for preparing it. You could say something like: "Marta, I'm really glad that you are supporting me and trying to help me with this program. It means a lot. I really care about you." Can you do that, Mike? Look right at her and give it a try.

CLIENT [Looking at his wife]: Marta, uh, I'm glad that you decided to give me another chance. I'm going to try to stay sober this time. [To therapist] What else?

THERAPIST: That was real good. What else might you add?

CLIENT: I'm glad you're giving me the Antabuse.

THERAPIST: There you go. Perfect. You did a very good job and it will get easier when I'm not watching you. You told her how you felt, why you felt it, and you thanked her for giving you the disulfiram.

Note: It is important for you to model the appropriate behavior, and to provide feedback to the couple after their attempt. Give positive reinforcement whenever possible, and shape the behavior as needed.

THERAPIST: Marta, what was it like to look at Mike and tell him how you felt?

WIFE: It felt real good. I mean, I thought I'd get angry. But instead it made me feel that maybe this time it will work. I'm not 100% convinced, though.

THERAPIST: It's just the first day, the first step. Mike, how did that make you feel inside?

CLIENT: Well, I felt pretty good. Like we're trying. She's giving me another chance. And even though I know she doesn't trust me totally, I bet she feels better by giving the disulfiram to me.

THERAPIST: Great. That's the way I hoped you'd feel. As time goes on, I want you to have a little dialogue about why you're taking the disulfiram, and how you feel every day when you take it. The important thing is to find one time during the day when you can always take it. Try to take it in the same place too. Make it a positive, daily ritual.

WIFE: Sure. We'll make time.

THERAPIST: Good. Good for you. And, Mike?

CLIENT: Does it matter if I take it in the night or in the day?

THERAPIST: It makes no difference, as long as you do it systematically, so you don't forget.

CLIENT: What do you think, Marta? Do it at night, right as we're getting into bed?

WIFE: Yeah, that would work.

Note: The therapist asks the couple about their feelings during the administration procedure, and has them select a convenient time for their daily ritual.

THERAPIST: OK. Now, let's go ahead, since we have had a dry run. The disulfiram is in front of you ready to go. I want you to pretend I'm not here. Turn your chairs facing each other and go through the whole process like you will at home.

CLIENT: Shouldn't we save it for tonight?

THERAPIST: No, take it right now. Go ahead, give it a try. And then bring it with you to each of our sessions, so I can see how you're doing with the procedure.

As stated earlier, there is no reason to delay the start of the disulfiram administration once a commitment has been made. If medically cleared, it is advisable to give the first dose before the client leaves the session. It also is important for the disulfiram to be brought to subsequent sessions and taken in your presence. It ensures that the client has a proper prescription, and that he or she is still willing to take it. It also provides an opportunity for you to observe the monitoring procedure, and to offer feedback and reinforcement.

♦ ♦

This chapter presented a complete description of the disulfiram component of the CRA program. Although it is considered an optional part of treatment, it appears strongly indicated in certain cases. There are many advantages to taking disulfiram, and these are best realized when the disulfiram administration procedure is followed exactly as described. But a disulfiram prescription is just one piece of the CRA package; one that typically is used only during the first 3 months of treatment. Given this, there are many other critical procedures described in the upcoming chapters that need to be incorporated into a comprehensive CRA program.

Appendix 4.A. *DISULFIRAM CONSENT*

I, the undersigned, accept disulfiram (Antabuse) therapy as a means of deterring myself from drinking alcoholic beverages. I recognize the dangers which are connected with drinking alcohol in any form, whether in beverages, cough mixtures, vitamin tonics or any other substance containing alcohol. I also realize that some other medications such as paraldehyde, metronidazole (Flagyl) or phenytoin (Dilantin) may cause problems. Therefore, any time a physician is prescribing for me I will tell him/her that I am taking disulfiram (Antabuse) so that (s)he can avoid giving me any other drug that might cause a bad reaction.

I understand that the reaction that occurs if a person drinks after taking disulfiram (Antabuse) is one involving much discomfort and sickness. This can include flushing of the face, sweating, throbbing in the head and neck, palpitations, breathing difficulty, nausea, vomiting, dizziness, blurring of vision and usually a significant fall in blood pressure. Whereas fatalities are uncommon, death could occur in someone who drinks while taking disulfiram (Antabuse).

For these reasons I will notify my family that I am taking this medication so that there will be no danger of my accidentally taking any alcohol. If I experience any unusual and persisting feelings or symptoms, I will contact my doctor so that (s)he can determine if they may be related to the medicine.

I fully understand that attempting to drink small amounts of alcohol while taking disulfiram (Antabuse) is a dangerous method of trying to control excessive drinking. Not only are there potentially dangerous physical effects, but the long-term effect may be to provoke a significant degree of emotional depression.

I understand that there is a possibility of a reaction which may last for many days (up to 14) after stopping disulfiram (Antabuse), should I take an alcoholic beverage thereafter. Should I want to commence taking disulfiram (Antabuse) again, I have to wait until all alcohol is out of my system before doing so (usually 24 hours from the time of the last drink).

Print Name of Client:_____

Signature of Client:_____

Date:_____

Signature of Witness:_____

Date:_____

APPENDIX 4.B   *SAMPLE LETTER TO PHYSICIAN*

(counselor's name)
Community Alcohol Program
123 High Street
Albuquerque, New Mexico 87111

Dear (physician's name):

   This letter is to inform you that (client's name) has agreed to take disulfiram to help control his/her urges to drink alcohol. The purpose of this referral is to have you medically evaluate his/her ability to take disulfiram. He/she has signed a voluntary Disulfiram Consent and has had the side effects of a disulfiram ethanol reaction explained in detail. The intent is to use disulfiram as an adjunct to his/her regular therapy program. It will be monitored by his/her_____.

   If you have any questions concerning (client's name) treatment program, please feel free to contact me. Enclosed please find a copy of the voluntary Disulfiram Consent, along with a Consent to Release Information.

Sincerely,

(counselor's name)_____
(counselor's title)_____

5

CRA Treatment Plan

At the time you begin to develop a treatment plan, you should have already examined the client's assessment instrument information, completed the functional analysis charts, conducted the Sobriety Sampling procedure, and presented the disulfiram option if applicable. This preparation enables you to guide the client through the treatment planning process using his or her own goals and reinforcers. CRA offers a set of procedures and forms to develop this comprehensive treatment plan, including the Happiness Scale and the Goals of Counseling. This chapter will introduce each component of the overall plan, and describe how to use it.

HAPPINESS SCALE

Description and Purpose

Having clients complete the Happiness Scale (Appendix 5.A) is the first step in the development of the treatment plan. The Happiness Scale is comprised of ten life categories: Drinking/Sobriety, Job or Educational Progress, Money Management, Social Life, Personal Habits, Marriage/ Family Relationships, Legal Issues, Emotional Life, Communication, and General Happiness. Clients are asked to rate each category on a scale of 1 (completely unhappy) to 10 (completely happy) to reflect how happy or satisfied they currently are with that area.

The Happiness Scale serves several important purposes: (1) It provides a precounseling baseline that indicates which areas of the client's life are in most need of immediate attention, (2) it motivates the client by pinpointing specific areas that require change, (3) it evaluates ongoing progress in therapy, and (4) it helps the client discriminate problem areas from nonproblem areas.

Explaining the Happiness Scale to a Client

The dialogue that follows shows a CRA therapist introducing the Happiness Scale to a client and providing a rationale. The instructions are next presented clearly. The therapist then checks that the client fully comprehends the task by doing the first few categories with him. The link between the client's drinking and his unhappiness in other life areas is pointed out when indicated.

THERAPIST: In order to come up with the best treatment plan for you, Charles, we need to first fill out a couple of forms. The first one is called the Happiness Scale. The purpose of this scale is to get a clear idea of how satisfied you are right now in all areas of your life . . . not just with your drinking. It will tell us which areas you feel you need to work on. I'll actually have you fill out one each session, so that we can monitor progress in each area. Does this make sense?

CLIENT: Yes . . . but what do I do?

THERAPIST: I'll go ahead and explain that right now. Let me show you the form.

Note: The therapist has given the rationale for the Happiness Scale. Now refer to Appendix 5.A.

THERAPIST: Do you see how there are ten categories listed here? The first nine represent specific areas of your life that we'll want to look at, such as #2, Job, and #4, Social Life. The last one, #10, is simply called General Happiness. We'll do that last because it stands for your overall satisfaction with your life once you take all the other nine areas into consideration. So let's go through this now, keeping in mind that you rate how happy you are *currently, today*, with each area.

I'd like you to use a 10-point rating scale. A rating of 1 means that you are completely unhappy with that part of your life now; about as unhappy as you could possibly be. A rating at the other end of the scale, a 10, means that you are completely happy with that area of your life. In other words, a 10 means that the particular area doesn't need any improvement or change whatsoever. You are satisfied with things in that area exactly the way they are. All the numbers between 1 and 10 represent less extreme versions of your happiness in an area. Ratings closer to 1 stand for relatively unhappy areas of your life, and ratings near the 10 end represent relatively happy areas. Let's do the first one together: Drinking/Sobriety. On this scale of 1 to 10, what rating represents how satisfied or how happy you are right now with that part of your life?

CLIENT: Oh, I suppose I'd have to give it a 2.

THERAPIST: That's fine. Now why don't you describe to me how you arrived at a 2, so I can be sure that you understand how the rating system is used.

CLIENT: I don't know what to do about that part of my life; I'm confused. I like to drink, but ever since I got that DWI I worry every time I have a beer. It's no fun anymore. But if I *don't* drink, my friends give me a hard time. And then I start to wonder if maybe they aren't the best friends to have!

THERAPIST: So it sounds like you're still confused about what you'd like to see happen with your drinking.

CLIENT: I don't even know if I'm confused! I mean, I know that I need to stop drinking. Too many bad things have happened lately that seem related to my drinking. So that's why I rated it a 2. I've got to do something about it.

THERAPIST: A rating of 2 means that you're just about as unhappy with that part of your life as you can imagine being. Does that sound right?

CLIENT: Yes, I would say so.

THERAPIST: Charles, in a few minutes we're going to set goals in each of these areas, and come up with ideas as to how you can reach your goals. But for now let's finish rating the items on the Happiness Scale. How satisfied are you with your job situation right now?

CLIENT: Not very. I'd rate it a 3.

THERAPIST: And what made you decide to rate it a 3? Again, that says that you're pretty unhappy with that part of your life.

Note: You may not know at this point whether the client's dissatisfaction with his job is related to being unemployed, to not enjoying his occupation or his work environment, or perhaps to not being content with his salary. In an effort to determine whether the rating is appropriate, you may need to inquire briefly about the nature of the dissatisfaction. Certainly this would become apparent later during the completion of the Goals of Counseling form.

CLIENT: Actually, I'm unhappy with my salary, not my job. I'm overdue for a raise, but I'm afraid to push it with my supervisor. You see, rumor has it that the boss is suspicious of my drinking. Maybe he started to wonder about all the extra sick days.

THERAPIST: Your rating suggests that this job situation bothers you a lot. Is that accurate?

CLIENT: I would have to say it does.

THERAPIST: It's interesting to see how these first two items on the Happiness Scale are actually related. I bet your job situation would improve if your drinking situation got better.

Note: Take the opportunity to point out the connection between the problem drinking and the client's dissatisfaction with other areas of his life.

THERAPIST: Go ahead and complete the ratings for the remaining eight items. Then I'll look it over to make sure that I'm following what you're telling me.

Note: Refer to Appendix 5.B for an example of a completed Happiness Scale.

Once a client has completed the Happiness Scale for the first time, you should review it briefly in its entirety. At times clients do not fully understand the instructions, and consequently circle all 1's. It is unlikely that a client will feel totally unhappy with every aspect of life. In the rare event that this occurs, problem solving (see Chapter 6) is used to help the client prioritize which problem to work on first. Occasionally a client will circle all 10's. You should test the hypothesis that this may represent a form of resistance.

Using the Happiness Scale Throughout Treatment

As mentioned earlier, information from the initial Happiness Scale can be very useful when formulating the treatment plan. This will become more apparent when its role with the Goals of Counseling form is illustrated in the next section. And once goals have been set in each area, progress can be monitored by having clients complete a new Happiness Scale at the start of each session. Regardless of whether the ratings increase or decrease in a category, it is important to investigate the reasons behind the noted changes that week. The behavior that contributed to the changes can then be either reinforced or discouraged.

In using the Happiness Scale to track progress, sometimes new difficulties are introduced. A client may consistently rate areas the same or lower as therapy proceeds. Although this may indicate a lack of progress in those areas, there are other possible explanations: (1) The client inadvertently modified his or her reference points on the scales over time as expectations changed. Consequently his or her interpretation of the entire rating system shifted as well. (2) The client's modified style of behaving caused Concerned Others to react in an unaccepting or uncomfortable manner that temporarily exaggerated relationship problems. Discuss these potential complications with clients early in therapy so that they will understand these reactions should they occur.

GOALS OF COUNSELING

Description and Purpose

The second step in developing a treatment plan is completing the Goals of Counseling form (Appendix 5.C) with the client. The same ten life areas that appeared on the Happiness Scale also are found on the Goals of Counseling form. The purpose of this form is to assist in setting specific goals for each of the client's major problem areas, and then to list the plan by which the client will attempt to alter the unwanted behaviors.

One of the advantages of using the Goals of Counseling form is that it highlights the fact that the problem drinking itself is only one of the areas requiring attention. Sometimes this becomes more apparent as therapy progresses, since underlying difficulties may surface once the drinking problem is removed. Many clients already are cognizant of these problems, and use the excessive drinking as a coping device.

Basic Rules for Completing the Goals of Counseling Form

The guidelines for completing the form are in line with CRA's overall positive approach. Clients must be taught to adhere to three basic rules when setting goals or specifying interventions:

1. Keep statements brief so that confusion is minimized.
2. Always state goals or strategies in a positive way. This means

you should indicate what you want and will do, as opposed to what you do *not* want and will *not* do.
3. Use only specific, measurable behaviors so that progress can be monitored readily.

Behavioral rehearsal and modeling may be utilized to help shape the client's behavior when filling out these forms. Rather than beginning with a client's most difficult problem areas, it is advisable to start with a category from the Happiness Scale for which the client indicated at least a fair amount of satisfaction. This enables the client to practice setting goals and devising interventions for more manageable problems first. Give the client several options from among the higher rated items, and allow him or her to select an area about which he or she feels most comfortable speaking.

The dialogue continues between Charles and his therapist. The Happiness Scale has been completed, and the basic rules for setting goals have been presented.

THERAPIST: We're ready to tackle your Goals of Counseling form now. I'd like to start with items from your Happiness Scale that you've rated relatively high. In other words, let's get some practice setting goals first with something a little more manageable. You gave higher ratings to Money Management, Social Life, Personal Habits, and Marriage or Family Relationships. Which one of these would you feel comfortable looking at first?

CLIENT: How about Social Life? What did I rate that?

THERAPIST: A 6. So that suggests there are some things you like about your social life, and some things you're not happy with. Let's talk about the parts you're dissatisfied with.

CLIENT: That's easy. I don't have a steady girlfriend, and I'd really like to. I date now and then, but they always seem to drink quite a bit. I'm starting to think that I should try to find someone who doesn't drink, or at least not a lot.

THERAPIST: You're off to a good start. Why don't you tell me in your own words what a reasonable goal would be to work toward?

CLIENT: I'm tired of dating women who drink all the time. I don't want to do it anymore.

THERAPIST: OK. So let's review our three basic rules and see if we need to fine-tune your goal a little. First, your statement was brief so you followed Rule #1. Did you state it in a positive way, though? I bet you could turn it around.

CLIENT: I'm not sure what you mean.

THERAPIST: How about, "I want to date women who don't drink."

CLIENT: Oh, I see. Make it sound like something good I'm *going* to do, as opposed to something I'm *not* going to do.

THERAPIST: Exactly. But before we write it on your form, let's see about Rule #3. Is it stated in specific terms? In other words, will we be able to measure whether you've accomplished your goal? Use actual numbers if you can.

CLIENT: Well, I can't really say that I'm going to go on a date once or twice a week, because I might ask someone who doesn't want to go. Then I wouldn't meet my goal, but it wouldn't really be my fault, right?

THERAPIST: True. So which behavior is under your control? We'll set a goal around that.

CLIENT: I think it would be good if I just got into the habit of asking out women who don't drink. That could be my goal. Then it wouldn't matter whether they turned me down.

THERAPIST: Great idea! Now let's hear it stated in a brief, positive, measurable way.

CLIENT: I'm going to ask out one woman a week who doesn't drink.

THERAPIST: Excellent! Let's write it down here under item #4.

The therapist shaped the client's vague initial goal into one that satisfied the three basic rules for goal setting. It is important to assist the client in this process, rather than doing it for him or her. Reinforce generously.

Determining an Appropriate Intervention

Once a goal has been set, assist the client in devising a reasonable plan for achieving that goal. The basic rules for specifying an intervention are the same as those listed for setting goals; namely, be brief, positive, and use specific (measurable) behaviors. Although some goals may require more than one intervention, be careful not to overwhelm the client with too many assignments at once. Be sure to indicate a time frame for each intervention in the final column of the Goals of Counseling form.

The dialogue continues between Charles and his therapist:

THERAPIST: Now our next step is to figure out a way that you're going to be able to accomplish your goal. We might be able to set things up so that you can do it on your own, or you might need some help from me; like for skills training of some sort. What do you think? How can we make sure that you'll be able to reach your goal?

CLIENT: Well, first I need to stop hanging out in bars all the time. That's not the best place to find someone who doesn't drink!

THERAPIST: Good point. So what do you need to do?

CLIENT: I'm not sure. I don't know where to go to meet women.

THERAPIST: Why don't we first review the nondrinking activities you enjoy, and see if any of them might provide an opportunity to meet available women. Here's your functional analysis for one nondrinking activity: Wednesday night dinner at your older brother's house. Remember what you liked about that?

CLIENT: Yes. My brother and his wife and kids treat me good. We usually play cards after dinner. And my older brother doesn't drink, so I never do there.

Note: The therapist refers to the client's CRA Functional Analysis for Nondrinking Behavior chart (discussed in Chapter 2) to get ideas for a sober social activity that potentially could involve meeting women.

THERAPIST: Is there any way these Wednesday night dinners could be used as an opportunity to meet new women?

CLIENT: Maybe. Actually my brother wanted to invite over a friend of his wife's a while back, but I asked him not to. It made me nervous. It felt too much like a blind date.

THERAPIST: So you don't want to pursue dinner at your brother's as one option for trying to meet your goal of asking out nondrinking women?

CLIENT: I didn't say that. I mean, you're right. A few months ago I would never have wanted to do it, but I feel different about things now.

THERAPIST: Great. So let's specify a brief, positive, measurable strategy.

Note: Just as with the goals, the intervention should be stated in brief, positive, and measurable terms.

CLIENT: I could do two things: First, I could make sure I go to my brother's house every Wednesday night. I started skipping weeks when I was drinking heavily again. And then I could be sure I mention to both my brother and his wife that I'm interested in meeting some nice women who don't drink.

THERAPIST: Sounds like a good plan. Here, I'll write it down. We need to specify a time frame, too. How often will you do each of these, and for how long?

CLIENT: I'll do them each week, on Wednesday night, and I imagine I'll just keep going to dinner there indefinitely.

THERAPIST: Fine. And for how long do you want to keep reminding them that you're anxious to meet a nondrinking female?

CLIENT (Laughs): I guess it could get pretty monotonous for me to remind them every week for months . . . even years! I'd have to start wondering about why they weren't inviting anyone over! How about I remind them weekly for a month?

Note: Refer to Appendix 5.D, item #4 for an example of how the therapist would be completing the Goals of Counseling form for this particular client and problem.

THERAPIST: Perfect. Let's keep going. You might need to come up with a second plan for meeting people, since we can't really rely on your brother to supply you with dates weekly. Any ideas?

CLIENT: Sometimes I like to hang out and read magazines at the coffee shop. I do it just to be out around people, but I could make a point of talking to some women who are there by themselves.

THERAPIST: Good plan. Can you be more specific?

CLIENT: Sure. I'll go to the Prairie Coffee Shop either Saturday or Sunday morning, and I'll strike up a conversation with at least one female stranger each time.

THERAPIST: And what about your time frame? You're already adding something new with your brother. Do you want to wait 2 weeks before starting this second plan?

Note: The therapist makes sure that the client is not accepting too many new intervention assignments for the upcoming week.

CLIENT: No, I think I can manage it all now. I almost always go to the coffee shop each weekend already. This would just be a matter of making sure I start a conversation.

THERAPIST: Fine. But you know, Charles, starting a conversation could be a long way off from your goal of asking someone out for a date. There are a lot of things that would need to happen in that conversation first before you ask anyone out.

CLIENT: True. But I could still say that my strategy is to talk to a new female. Only if it seems appropriate will I ask her out. I mean, I wouldn't ask her out without having a decent conversation first. And then if I just kept it real casual, like maybe meeting her later that week for coffee again, it wouldn't really even seem like an official date.

THERAPIST: OK. You've convinced me! I'll add that to your Goals of Counseling form, too, then. But I'm also going to note in parentheses that we will practice role-plays in the event that you feel dissatisfied with how your conversations have been going there after a month.

If the therapist had remained concerned that her client did not have the social skills to start and carry an appropriate conversation, she immediately would have had the client role-play the situation. Behavioral rehearsal and feedback are often critical components of these plans. Regardless, it would be important to check with the client at the next session to determine the status of the planned strategies. Unanticipated difficulties could be role-played and corrected.

Planning for Skills Training

Frequently the appropriate intervention or plan for addressing a specific problem involves a skill that the client does not possess. Early in therapy you may simply have to note the appropriate CRA procedure on the Goals of Counseling form, and indicate the time frame for teaching the skill. Some therapists find it useful to place parentheses around interventions that require their direct assistance, whether it involves straightforward behavioral rehearsal or the complete training of a new skill. It serves as a quick reminder of CRA procedures that still need to be taught.

In the continuing dialogue between Charles and his therapist a second problem area will be addressed. This time the need for skills training will be obvious. Note that the therapist now puts increased responsibility on Charles to set the goal and design an intervention.

THERAPIST: I'm going to give you a copy of this Goals of Counseling form. That way you can remind yourself, if you need to, about what you've agreed to work on, and how you planned to accomplish each goal. Now let's practice setting one more manageable goal today. Which of the higher rated areas would you like to tackle next?

CLIENT: Let's try a 7 this time: Marriage and Family Relationships.

THERAPIST: A fine choice. Now, this time I'm going to leave the whole goal-setting process more up to you. What do you do first?

CLIENT: I'd like to talk about my relationship with my younger brother, Oliver. Sometimes we get along really well, and sometimes it's a complete disaster. But let's see . . . I need to come up with a goal.

THERAPIST: Right. And in stating your goal you are going to remember to be what?

CLIENT: Brief, specific, and positive.

THERAPIST: Very good . . . as long as you remember that "specific" means measurable.

Note: The therapist makes certain that the client remembers the three rules for setting goals and naming interventions.

CLIENT: I want to say that my goal is to get along better with Oliver, but that doesn't give you anything to measure.

THERAPIST: No, but it *is* stated in a brief and positive way, so you're on the right track.

Note: The therapist uses every opportunity to reinforce the client.

CLIENT: This one's complicated, because I really have to set a goal to see Oliver first, before I set one about how I'm going to act toward him. You see, I've been avoiding him lately because he hassles me about my drinking, and at the same time he almost pushes beer at me whenever we're together.

THERAPIST: It's interesting how so many of these other problems are connected with your drinking pattern.

Note: As stated earlier, you should outline the association between a client's drinking and the reported nondrinking problem areas whenever possible.

THERAPIST: Do you think, though, that he'll stop hassling you now that you're actively working on your drinking problem?

CLIENT: No, because he'll harp on all the "horrible things" drinking has already done to me, and how my life is a waste. And then he'll try to tempt me with a bottle. He's done it before.

THERAPIST: It sounds like maybe we need to figure out a way for you to let Oliver know that you're really not interested in drinking, and that he needs to stop bringing up problems from the past.

CLIENT: But I've tried to do that already. It doesn't work. Don't get me wrong, though, Oliver's still a good guy. He just upsets me when he starts in with this sort of thing.

Note: It is clear to the therapist at this point that the client needs some skills training to effectively work toward a goal in the family relationship area. Depending on the time frame established for this problem, you may elect to either introduce skills training now, or to set an appointment for a later date. This plan should be listed in parentheses on the "Intervention" section of the Goals of Counseling form, since the relevant CRA techniques have not been taught yet.

THERAPIST: I know your brother means a lot to you, and so that's a good reason to learn a better way to deal with him when he starts to give you a hard time. I plan on showing you a technique that's designed specifically to let people know you're serious about not drinking, and one that's intended to teach you how to communicate more effectively in general. So don't worry yet about *how* you're going to accomplish your goals in the family relationship area. Let's just go ahead and set some first.

Note: The therapist introduces the notion of drink-refusal and communication skills training, but decides to get clear goals established before proceeding with any further explanation of them.

CLIENT: OK. The first goal has to do with just seeing more of Oliver. So I'll say that I'm going to invite him over to watch TV once every other week on a weeknight.

THERAPIST: Your goal sounds brief, positive, and measurable, so that's excellent. Now, I remember, though, from your functional analysis that watching TV was a high-risk drinking activity. Wasn't it?

Note: The therapist reinforces the client, and then ties in relevant information from his functional analysis.

CLIENT: Actually, I wouldn't connect all TV watching with drinking, just sports shows. Boy oh boy, did we ever get wasted during football season.

THERAPIST: But do you think it's a good idea to select watching TV as your first activity with your brother? He may still try to tempt you with alcohol at first.

CLIENT: I think it will be OK. I'm already watching TV without drinking when I'm alone. How about if I just make sure we do it at my place since I don't have any alcohol there. And Oliver would never bring any over . . . he's too cheap!

THERAPIST: It's sounding better all the time.

Note: See Appendix 5.D, item #6A.

THERAPIST: Let's talk about your intervention. What's your plan for reaching this goal?

CLIENT: I'll call him tonight, while I'm still thinking about it. I'll ask him what his favorite TV night is, and then see if he wants to stop by then.

THERAPIST: Charles, you're doing a terrific job. Let's go ahead with the next goal in this problem area. You said something about wanting to get along with Oliver better.

CLIENT: Yes. I don't want to get into any arguments with him about my drinking. I don't want to listen to him about the problems it's caused, and I don't want to get into a screaming match if he tries to give me beer.

Simplifying a Complicated Goal

It is common for a goal to actually involve a number of components. Tackling such a goal will feel less overwhelming to the client if you help him or her break down the goal into several smaller, more manageable ones. In this way the interventions usually are more obvious. The therapist assists Charles in this process.

THERAPIST: Let's simplify this by breaking it into two goals. What would you like to work toward with regard to the first part of the goal: listening to him talk about the problems your drinking has caused?

CLIENT: I would like to be able to calmly stop him if he brings up the subject.

THERAPIST: Now you're getting there! How about our three rules?

Note: The therapist is helping to shape the client's response into a clear goal that is brief, positive, and measurable.

CLIENT: Let's see. It's brief, and I guess it's positive. I'll add that I'll do this every time he brings up the subject. There. It's measurable now, too.

THERAPIST: I'll add this to the form. Let's come up with your plan for accomplishing this.

CLIENT: I don't know what to say here, because like I said, everything I've tried ends up in a fight.

THERAPIST: So that means we need to work on skills that allow you to speak to your brother assertively. It involves some basic rules to follow, and then role-plays. So I'll add that on the form. I'm putting my part in parentheses. For a time frame, how about we say that I'll start working on communication skills training with you next week. We'll plan to practice it for a month. OK. How should we state the second part of the goal; the one that concerns your brother offering you alcohol?

CLIENT: Actually it's pretty similar. I want to be able to just tell him I'm not interested. Period.

THERAPIST: Good. So I'll list it the same way as the last one. Do you think you'll need some practice in figuring out the best way to tell him you're not interested?

CLIENT: Definitely.

THERAPIST: Then I'll put that we'll practice drink refusal. It's another skill, but in some ways it's similar to communication skills training. We really can cover both types of training in the same sessions, so I'll note the same time frame, too. Now that's plenty for today!

Note: Refer to Appendix D, items 6B and C. The remainder of the Goals of Counseling form has been completed as well, in order to serve as a model.

Although the Goals of Counseling form typically is completed during the first or second session, at times part of it may be assigned as homework. In the latter case, be sure to cover one or two areas thoroughly so that the client has a guide from which to work. Then be cautious not to overwhelm the client by assigning too many categories. The current example involved a high-functioning client who demonstrated during the session that he was capable of attempting a fair amount of the work on his own. Consequently the therapist would feel comfortable assigning a sizable homework task, such as filling in one goal and intervention for each remaining category. It would be reviewed in its entirety at the next session, and modified when necessary.

The Goals of Counseling form should be reexamined at least once a month throughout the treatment program. Give the client recognition for goals that were achieved, and reinforce the person for efforts that were made. If certain problem areas have goals that have not been reached for more than several weeks, the interventions should be reviewed to determine their appropriateness, and possibly to refine them. This is also an excellent time for the client to add new goals.

Potential Problems in Completing the Goals of Counseling Form

The dialogue between the therapist and Charles illustrated most of the common difficulties encountered when attempting to complete the Goals of Counseling form:

1. Actually applying the three basic rules to "real-life" problems. Most individuals seem to naturally talk about their problems in terms that are vague, negative, and nonmeasurable.
2. Designing goals and interventions that are too complex, and consequently are confusing and difficult to follow.

3. Leaving out important steps that are necessary in working toward certain goals.
4. Including plans that really are not under the client's own control.
5. Unnecessarily placing oneself in a high-risk drinking situation.

In addition to these common problems, occasionally you may find yourself working with clients who are opposed to spending time addressing any nondrinking problem areas. Their belief is that once they stop drinking, the other problems automatically will disappear. Although the problems rarely get resolved in this manner, the CRA therapist usually will allow clients to discover this through experience, and consequently will work with them exclusively on their drinking problem first.

♦ ♦

Thus far this book has focused on the assessment and treatment plan development phases of therapy. The next chapter begins the presentation of the CRA skills training procedures more commonly associated with the treatment segment of therapy. You will notice, however, that assessment and treatment planning actually play significant roles for the duration of the therapy process.

Appendix 5.A   *HAPPINESS SCALE*

This scale is intended to estimate your *current* happiness with your life in each of the ten areas listed. You are to circle one of the numbers (1–10) beside each area. Numbers toward the left end of the 10-unit scale indicate various degrees of unhappiness, while numbers toward the right end of the scale reflect increasing levels of happiness. Ask yourself this question as you rate each life area: "How happy am I *with this area of my life*?" In other words, state according to the numerical scale (1–10) exactly how you feel today. Try to exclude all feelings of yesterday and concentrate only on the feelings of today in each of the life areas. Also try *not* to allow one category to influence the results of the other categories.

	Completely unhappy									Completely happy
1. Drinking/Sobriety	1	2	3	4	5	6	7	8	9	10
2. Job or Educational Progress	1	2	3	4	5	6	7	8	9	10
3. Money Management	1	2	3	4	5	6	7	8	9	10
4. Social Life	1	2	3	4	5	6	7	8	9	10
5. Personal Habits	1	2	3	4	5	6	7	8	9	10
6. Marriage/Family Relationships	1	2	3	4	5	6	7	8	9	10
7. Legal Issues	1	2	3	4	5	6	7	8	9	10
8. Emotional Life	1	2	3	4	5	6	7	8	9	10
9. Communication	1	2	3	4	5	6	7	8	9	10
10. General Happiness	1	2	3	4	5	6	7	8	9	10

Name:_____

Date:_____

Appendix 5.B *HAPPINESS SCALE*

This scale is intended to estimate your *current* happiness with your life in each of the ten areas listed. You are to circle one of the numbers (1–10) beside each area. Numbers toward the left end of the 10-unit scale indicate various degrees of unhappiness, while numbers toward the right end of the scale reflect increasing levels of happiness. Ask yourself this question as you rate each life area: "How happy am I *with this area of my life*?" In other words, state according to the numerical scale (1–10) exactly how you feel today. Try to exclude all feelings of yesterday and concentrate only on the feelings of today in each of the life areas. Also try *not* to allow one category to influence the results of the other categories.

	Completely unhappy									Completely happy
1. Drinking/Sobriety	1	(2)	3	4	5	6	7	8	9	10
2. Job or Educational Progress	1	2	(3)	4	5	6	7	8	9	10
3. Money Management	1	2	3	4	5	(6)	7	8	9	10
4. Social Life	1	2	3	4	5	(6)	7	8	9	10
5. Personal Habits	1	2	3	4	5	6	(7)	8	9	10
6. Marriage/Family Relationships	1	2	3	4	5	6	(7)	8	9	10
7. Legal Issues	1	2	(3)	4	5	6	7	8	9	10
8. Emotional Life	1	2	3	4	(5)	6	7	8	9	10
9. Communication	1	2	3	4	(5)	6	7	8	9	10
10. General Happiness	1	2	3	(4)	5	6	7	8	9	10

Name: *Charles*

Date: *6/1*

APPENDIXES 5.C–5.D

Appendix 5.C   GOALS OF COUNSELING   Name: _____   Date: _____

Problem Areas/Goals	Intervention	Time Frame
1. In the area of drinking/sobriety I would like:		
2. In the area of job/educational progress I would like:		
3. In the area of money management I would like:		
4. In the area of social life I would like:		
5. In the area of personal habits I would like:		

Problem Areas/Goals	Intervention	Time Frame
6. In the area of marriage/family relationships I would like:		
7. In the area of legal issues I would like:		
8. In the area of emotional life I would like:		
9. In the area of communication I would like:		
10. In the area of general happiness I would like:		

Appendix 5.D   GOALS OF COUNSELING   Name: _Charles_   Date: _6/1_

Problem Areas/Goals	Intervention	Time Frame
1. In the area of drinking/sobriety I would like: _To stay abstinent for 90 days._	_(1) Attend weekly therapy. (2) (Problem-Solving Training) to address difficulties with staying abstinent as they arise._ _(3) (Drink-Refusal Training). (4) Start taking Antabuse daily with a monitor (older bro.) if I drink any alcohol during the next week. (Therapist will check at next session)._	_(6/1–9/1); weekly (6/8–7/8)_ _weekly (6/8–7/1)_ _check 6/8_
2. In the area of job/educational progress I would like: _To get a 5% raise over the next yr. (2 1/2% ea. 6 months)._	_(1) Don't call in sick anymore . . . even if there's been a drinking episode. (2) (Assertiveness Training) regarding how to approach my boss for a raise._ _(3) Present myself to my boss and ask for a raise._	_(6/1–12/1)_ _(11/1–12/1)_ _12/1_
3. In the area of money management I would like: _To learn how to budget my money better so I can pay my monthly bills on time._	_(1) Meet with my sister-in-law one evening so she can show me how she budgets her family's income._ _(2) Figure out how much money I typically spent on alcohol ea. wk. Determine what I can now use that money for._	_by 6/15_ _by 6/15_
4. In the area of social life I would like: _To ask out one woman a wk. who doesn't drink._	_(1) Go to bro.'s house for dinner every Weds. night._ _(2) Tell bro. & his wife that I'd like to meet a nice woman who doesn't drink. (3) Go to Prairie Coffee Shop every Sat. or Sun. AM. (4) Talk to at least one female stranger ea. time._ _(5) Practice role-plays with therapist if necessary)._	_weekly (6/1–?)_ _weekly (6/1–7/1)_ _weekly (6/1–?)_ _weekly (6/1–7/1)_ _check 7/1_
5. In the area of personal habits I would like: _To keep my car clean inside and out: washed & vacuumed once/wk. & waxed bimonthly._	_(1) (Problem-Solving Training) - to figure out a way around all the obstacles to getting this task done._ _(2) (Check on progress)._	_7/1_ _weekly (7/8–8/8)_

Problem Areas/Goals	Intervention	Time Frame
6. In the area of marriage/family/relationships I would like: A. To invite Oliver over to watch TV once every other wk. B. To be able to calmly stop him every time he brings up the subject of probs. my drinking has caused. C. To be able to calmly stop him every time he offers me alcohol by telling him I'm not interested in drinking.	A. (1) Call Oliver & see what his favorite TV night is. Invite over. B. (1) (Communication Skills Training) C. (1) (Drink-Refusal Training)	6/1 biweekly (6/1–?) weekly (6/8–7/8) weekly (6/8–7/8)
7. In the area of legal issues I would like: A. To have a clean legal record from now on. B. To pay off my legal fines.	A. (1) Only drive when I've had nothing to drink. B. (1) [see #3: Money Management] (2) Use the money I've saved from projected alcohol expenses this 1st month to pay off my DWI fine.	(6/1–?) 6/15 7/1
8. In the area of emotional life I would like: To find 1–2 close male friends who don't drink daily.	(1) Identify a list of 10 non-alcohol-related social activities. (2) (Systematic Encouragement & Reinforcer Sampling) to assure compliance. (3) Try one new non-alcohol-related social activity ea. wk. (4) (Problem-Solve) for difficulties that arise during these activities.	(6/1–6/8) (6/8–7/8) (6/8–8/8) (6/8–8/8)
9. In the area of communication I would like: To be able to talk to my parents in a calm, friendly way without arguing.	(1) (Problem-Solving Training) to figure out the 10 "safest" topics to discuss. (2) (Communication Skill Training) to know how to calmly switch topics, etc. if an argument starts to develop.	6/15 weekly (6/22–7/22)
10. In the area of general happiness I would like: A. To feel satisfied with my job performance. B. To have a few close male & female friends who don't drink. C. To feel comfortable meeting socially with my parents & brothers.	A. [see #2]. B. [see #4 & 8]. C. [see #6 & 9].	by 12/1 by 9/1 by 8/1

6

Behavioral Skills Training

Behavioral skills training has been incorporated into the treatment of several substance abuse disorders over the years, including alcohol (Monti, Abrams, Kadden, & Cooney, 1989), cannabis (Hawkins, Catalano, Gillmore, & Wells, 1989), and more recently cocaine dependence (Childress et al., 1993). Since its inception, CRA has viewed skills training as an essential treatment ingredient. This chapter will describe a combination of original CRA skills training procedures and successful techniques adapted from other researchers' work.

COMMUNICATION SKILLS TRAINING

One fundamental deficiency of many alcohol-abusing clients is the inability to communicate in a positive, effective manner. Interestingly, the majority of these individuals are unaware of even having communication difficulties. You may need to illustrate their problem by giving concrete examples of conversations that are either too aggressive or too passive. Motivate these clients to work on this behavior by pointing out that speaking in a positive, assertive manner will increase the probability of having their needs met.

According to CRA, effective communication can be broken down into three basic parts: (1) giving an understanding statement, (2) taking partial responsibility, and (3) offering to help. An understanding statement introduces feelings into the discussion, particularly empathy. A partial responsibility statement indicates that the client is willing to accept a role in creating or solving a specific problem. A final way to enhance a conversation is through an offer to help. Taken together these components deliver a message of wanting a change, but with a willingness on the part of the requester to be actively supportive in the process. The outcome is a decrease in the defensiveness of the individual being addressed, and open lines of communication.

We will demonstrate each type of statement in a dialogue. The conversation that follows between a therapist and his client, Marlene, involves making a request of another person. The discussion centers around Marlene's desire to ask her boyfriend to accompany her to a few therapy sessions. She is quite certain that he will be reluctant to do so. Nevertheless, both Marlene and the therapist believe that Paul's involvement in her therapy is important right now. The dialogue begins with the therapist evaluating Marlene's basic communication skill level during a role-play. Gradually he will introduce the relevant CRA conversation enhancers.

THERAPIST: Let's do a role-play of your conversation with Paul when you're first asking him to accompany you to a session. I'll play Paul's part.

Start off by asking him the question in the way you normally would, and then I'll give you ideas about how to make it a more positive conversation.

CLIENT: OK. Paul, remember I told you I was going to see a therapist about my drinking?

THERAPIST [playing boyfriend]: Oh, right. That again. You went to see another therapist. Well, what did this one say?

CLIENT: Lot's of interesting things. I think I have a good chance of succeeding this time, but I could use your help.

THERAPIST [playing boyfriend]: Here it comes! So this time your doctor wants to drag me in on it?

CLIENT (An aside to the therapist): Uh-oh. Here's where I get nervous.

THERAPIST: Just tell him what you'd like him to do, and why it's important. I'll play him giving you a hard time still, so I can show you some other important parts of a good conversation.

Note: The therapist is assessing the client's basic communication skill level during these initial interchanges. He will introduce the specific CRA communication enhancers as needed.

CLIENT: I'd like you to come to a few therapy sessions with me. It might help me and our relationship, too.

THERAPIST [playing boyfriend]: Well, it seems silly for me to make a big deal out of this one way or the other, since I have the feeling we're only talking about a week or so. Let's face it, Marlene, you lose your enthusiasm for these programs pretty quickly.

CLIENT [an aside to the therapist]: Help! This is where it usually turns into an argument.

THERAPIST: Perfect. Then this is where we need to try something new. Start in by making an understanding statement. Do you know what I mean? Explain how you see where he's coming from. It usually helps to think of a time when you were in a similar situation. You may even want to mention it.

Note: The therapist introduces the idea of adding an understanding statement to the request. This should enable the boyfriend to feel validated for being hesitant to get involved.

CLIENT: Paul, I can understand why you're so skeptical. I remember being real skeptical about my friend Rose's commitment to lose weight. She tried every fad diet that came out. It was hard to keep getting enthusiastic with her each time something new appeared on the market. [An aside to the therapist] Great . . . now he's never going to want to do it.

THERAPIST: But we're not done yet! You're off to a good start, though. I can almost guarantee that he'll be listening carefully to you now, because you've convinced him that you're trying to understand what it feels like to him. Now it's time to accept partial responsibility for the problem or for the solution.

Note: Here the therapist instructs the client to add the second component of a good communication: a partial responsibility statement. Typically this softens the request.

CLIENT: Partial responsibility? Isn't it *all* my fault?

THERAPIST: Well, I could argue with you on that, but it really comes down to what we're calling the problem. The problem we're dealing with now is Paul's reluctance to sincerely support your efforts to stay sober by being involved in your treatment program. Now you don't want to start blaming him for never being supportive. I imagine you could have quite a disagreement over that issue.

CLIENT: I see what you mean. You're right. We've been there before. OK. So I should accept partial responsibility for his attitude about this right now. How about this: Paul, I imagine it would be a lot easier for you to agree to this if I hadn't already dropped out of treatment a couple of times. It would mean a lot to me, though, because I care so much about you.

THERAPIST: Wow . . . you're getting fancy there! You accepted partial responsibility for his predicament, and you even shared your feelings. Excellent work. The third specific thing I'd like you to add to this positive communication is an offer to help. Can you think of something you could offer to do that would make it easier for him to agree to be involved?

CLIENT: Let's see. I suppose I could offer to drive. I could stop by his house before the session to pick him up. And maybe I could treat him to a coffee or something afterwards.

THERAPIST: I like the idea. You'd both be doing something nice for each other.

The therapist would have the client practice several versions of this role-play. This would prepare her for a wide range of possible reactions from her boyfriend. Then an assignment would be made to actually have a similar conversation with her boyfriend in the upcoming week. The therapist would review the outcome at the next session.

You should note that although the dialogue illustrated the usefulness of the three CRA communication components when making a request, there are many other relevant applications. Virtually any type of problem situation can be discussed more effectively between two individuals within such a framework. Simply be sure to have your client role-play several variations of this positive communication procedure, so that its generalizability becomes obvious. Then assign homework to attempt a positive conversation at home or work about a preplanned topic. Check on the progress in the subsequent session.

PROBLEM-SOLVING TRAINING

A second basic skill that is valuable for addressing a wide range of difficult behaviors or situations is problem solving. The main purpose of the problem-solving procedure for alcohol- abusing clients is to teach them strategies for coping with the daily hassles of their environment without returning to alcohol or drug use. But CRA does not stop with the introduction of a new technique. It also teaches clients to conceptualize all of their difficulties, no matter how seemingly insurmountable, as problems simply requiring a workable solution. This problem-solving orientation is generalized to fit many different kinds of dilemmas, and not necessarily only those related to substance abuse. The training prepares clients to be self-sufficient when formal therapy ends.

Problem-Solving Steps

Within the CRA format a modified version of the problem-solving approach originally introduced by D'Zurilla and Goldfried (1971) is utilized. The steps are as follows:

A. *Defining the Problem*
  1. Define the problem as specifically as possible.
  2. Separate out any secondary or related problems.

B. *Generating Alternatives*
  1. Use brainstorming to generate potential solutions.
  2. Do not criticize any of the suggestions offered.
  3. Go for quantity; the more potential solutions, the better!
  4. Stay within the problem area.
  5. State solutions in specific terms.

C. *Deciding on a Solution*
  1. Eliminate any solutions that you would not feel comfortable attempting. No explanations are needed.
  2. Evaluate the feasibility of each remaining alternative while identifying its probable consequences.
  3. Decide on one solution and describe exactly how you will carry it out.
  4. Consider possible obstacles to enacting the solution.
  5. Generate "backup" plans to circumvent these obstacles.
  6. Commit to trying the selected solution an agreed-upon number of times before the next session.
  7. Decide whether to attempt a second solution as well.
  8. Go through steps 2-6 of Deciding on a Solution for each subsequent solution considered.

D. *Evaluating the Outcome*
  1. Review the outcome at the next session and give a satisfaction rating.
  2. Modify the solution if necessary.
  3. If an entire new solution is required, repeat the problem-solving procedure.

CRA therapists often present this information to clients by outlining the steps on a board, or giving the clients a photocopy of a handout and having them follow along. Questions are encouraged throughout. Once you have explained the process, it is time to illustrate the problem-solving procedure with a real problem.

Begin by asking your client to mention a few current problems that he or she would like to address. If necessary, refer to the client's Goals of Counseling form for ideas. Select a problem that appears relatively specific and uncomplicated. Demonstrate step-by-step the problem-solving procedure with this real problem. Solicit the client's input throughout, but assist generously. You may elect to write the responses for each step on the board.

The dialogue that follows is an example of problem-solving training. Assume the therapist has already outlined the steps of the technique, and is ready to illustrate it with a current problem.

THERAPIST: Evelyn, earlier today you said you were concerned about your inability to fall asleep at night. In the past you've relied on two or three drinks before bedtime to help. Does this sound like a problem you'd like to work on?

CLIENT: Big time. I always have trouble sleeping, even if I drink.

THERAPIST: Let's make sure we both know exactly what your sleep problem is. Go ahead and describe it. I'll be writing down significant parts on the board.

CLIENT: I just can't fall asleep. My mind keeps racing. Once I fall asleep I'm usually OK. But it seems like it takes forever. I just can't seem to relax.

THERAPIST: It sounds like you're really having a miserable time with it. I've jotted all those things down. Can you make it any more specific, like maybe saying how often this happens?

CLIENT: Pretty much every night.

Note: The therapist helps the client begin Step A: Defining the Problem. Refer to Appendix 6.A for a simulated blackboard presentation of this problem-solving session.

THERAPIST: Now let's see if we can identify any obvious related problems. Evelyn, are there any things going on that might directly contribute to your sleep problem? Is there too much noise or light?

CLIENT: Not really. I live alone and my bedroom is just the way I want it.

THERAPIST: Why don't you describe to me your activities from suppertime until bedtime. Include any smoking, drinking, food, and other activities.

CLIENT: I usually eat at a fast-food place on the way home from work; usually a burger and a Coke. I go home, make a pot of coffee, watch TV until the news is over, and then go to bed around eleven o'clock. Oh yeah, I smoke about 10 to 15 cigarettes. I used to go to a bar a couple of nights a week. But I'm not drinking now, so I just stay home.

THERAPIST: Are there any other activities that you do at night?

CLIENT: No, not really. Sometimes a friend stops by, but not so much since I stopped drinking.

THERAPIST: There are several things I should point out. Your sleep problem may be partly due to your lifestyle. Both Coke and coffee have caffeine in them. Caffeine is a stimulant. Cigarettes contain nicotine, which is also a stimulant. Sitting in front of the TV most of the night doesn't promote good sleep habits either. We should keep these in mind when we start to come up with possible solutions. I'll put them on the blackboard under Related Problems as a reminder.

Note: The therapist has completed both sections of the first step. She is ready to start Step B: Generating Alternatives.

THERAPIST: Our next step is where we come up with possible solutions. You might remember I called it brainstorming. So let's get creative and see how long a list we can make. But like I explained earlier, one of the rules of brainstorming is that every suggestion by either of us gets put on the board. It doesn't matter if it sounds like something you'd never do, or if it's something you've already tried that doesn't work. We'll worry about that later. So no criticism here. The more potential solutions, the better! Just try to be specific, and make sure it's related to your sleep problem.

CLIENT: A friend once told me about some tea that makes you sleep better. How about that?

THERAPIST: Good, Evelyn. Sleepytime tea. That's a good start. What else could you do?

CLIENT: Exercise, I suppose. Like go for a walk. I guess I could cut down on my smoking and coffee at night, too.

THERAPIST: Great, now you're on track. What else?

CLIENT: I'm out of ideas. Is there something else?

THERAPIST: Since we're just generating ideas I'll throw in a few. Some people find that taking a hot bath is very relaxing, or reading a book just before bedtime. Other clients of mine have had luck with relaxation tapes or meditation. Do you think you could come up with just a few more?

CLIENT: OK. I could drink and take Valium again [*laughs*]. Just kidding.

THERAPIST: I'm glad. But just to show you this can be fun, let's put them up there. I'm counting on your not selecting them, though!

CLIENT: How about listen to quiet music? That might help.

Note: The therapist has completed the Generating Alternatives section, and is ready to move on to Step C: Deciding on a Solution.

THERAPIST: It's time to make some decisions now. Take a look at the list of possible solutions we generated. Go ahead and cross out any that you know won't work for you, or that you're definitely not interested in trying. Remember that I'm not allowed to ask any questions here. You don't need to explain your reasons for crossing them out.

CLIENT: I really don't think I want to try the hot bath, the book, or the meditation. And of course, I'm not going to pick the drinking or the Valium.

THERAPIST: Fine. Now look at the remaining ones. Think about what it would be like to try to carry them out. Do you think you'd do it? Would they work? You may end up eliminating more this way.

CLIENT: I'm going to drop the music one because I've had trouble actually getting myself to do it in the past. And I don't have the money for a relaxation tape right now.

THERAPIST: Good. Now pick one solution to start off. Evelyn, which one can you picture yourself doing several times this week?

CLIENT: I'd like to try that tea at night. And then I'd automatically cut down on my coffee, too. I'd like to just eliminate it completely after dinner.

THERAPIST: Sounds good. Now describe exactly how you'll do it. For instance, when will you buy the tea?

CLIENT: On my way home today. And I'll leave it sitting on my counter so I remember to use it.

THERAPIST: Can you think of anything that might get in the way of your being able to get or use the Sleepytime tea, or to cut down on the coffee?

Note: The therapist is attempting to identify any obstacles that might interfere with completing the assignment. In this manner these potential problems can be addressed in advance.

CLIENT: No. I have enough money for the tea, and I've even seen it in the store. No . . . I can do those.

THERAPIST: And what happens if the store is out of the tea today? What's your backup plan?

CLIENT: I know of another store across town that carries a lot of teas and coffee. I could call there to see if they have it. I know they'll at least have some kind of decaffeinated tea.

THERAPIST: Good. And how many times will you use the tea in the up-coming week?

Note: The therapist first checks on the backup plan, and then makes sure there is no question about the number of times the solution will be tried that week.

CLIENT: I'm going to try to use the tea every night. No, I'd better say five times this week. And those are the nights I won't drink coffee. I may not be home this weekend, so that could mess up the plan if I say seven nights.

THERAPIST: I'm convinced that you've got a good, solid plan. Now, we can either leave it like this or add one or two more potential solutions.

CLIENT: I'd really like to do more. This sleep thing has been bugging me a lot. How about I cut down to five cigarettes after dinner, too?

THERAPIST: Do you think you can do it? Picture yourself only having five cigarettes after dinner. Is it a realistic goal? What would be the consequences of trying to cut down to five?

Note: The therapist is now going through Steps 2–6 of C: Deciding on a Solution with this second solution.

CLIENT: Maybe I should say eight. That sounds better. I'm afraid I couldn't stick to five.

THERAPIST: Fine. Now comes the part where you tell me exactly how you're going to do it.

CLIENT: If I only bring eight home from work, I'll only smoke eight. I'll remember to do that. I've often thought of cutting back on the number I bring home.

THERAPIST: What might get in the way of your only bringing eight cigarettes home? This sounds like a crucial part of your solution.

CLIENT: It is. Let's see. I'll write it on my daily calendar. I always check that before I leave work. And if for some reason I don't, I'll give them to my neighbor as soon as I discover them.

Note: The therapist encourages the client to consider possible obstacles. The client offers backup plans as well.

THERAPIST: And how many times this week will you only smoke eight cigarettes after dinner?

CLIENT: Five times will be good for that one, too; the weeknights.

Note: Again the therapist has the client commit to an agreed-upon number of times to try the new solution before the next session.

THERAPIST: Good luck, Evelyn! At your next session we'll do the last part of problem solving where we go over the solutions you tried for the week. If you've done them and they've worked . . . great! But we may need to change them a little so they work even better. Let's not worry about that for now, though.

It is essential to introduce Step D: Evaluating the Outcome, at the next session. In the process, be sure to reinforce the client's efforts. Modify any solutions that did not work well, or that your client had great difficulty completing. In the event that your client did not even attempt to do the assignment, you may decide to identify the lack of follow-through as a problem needing attention. The entire problem-solving procedure could be devoted to it.

Once your client appears to fully understand the technique, have him or her take you through the entire procedure step-by-step with a new problem. This level of skill ultimately will be required before the client terminates treatment.

DRINK-REFUSAL TRAINING

Drink-refusal training is the third basic skill area that will be described in this chapter. CRA's version of drink-refusal training has four components: (1) enlisting the support of family and friends, (2) reviewing identified high-risk situations, (3) learning to refuse drinks assertively, and (4) restructuring negative thoughts.

Enlisting Social Support

One basic premise of CRA is that individuals will continue to engage in activities for which they receive reinforcement from their social environment. With this in mind, it seems logical to have motivated alcohol-abusing clients surround themselves with individuals supportive of sobriety.

As a first step in enlisting social support, have your client inform several family members and friends about the decision to stop drinking. Most clients expect to get mixed reactions to this announcement, ranging from pleasure and praise to disbelief and anger. Regardless of the response, clients should make it clear that they need to have their decision respected, and that they would appreciate the support of friends and family. Role-plays of these interactions are recommended.

In the course of practicing role-plays it is useful to pursue the issue of some people being uncomfortable when the client first stops drinking. Reassure your client that these individuals usually relax after they have grown accustomed to this new behavior. To help them adapt to the situation, instruct your client to be consistent about refusing alcohol, without making it an issue. Your client also would be well-advised not to be judgmental of friends who still drink. Drinking or not drinking is a personal decision, and mutual respect for each other's decision is the basis for maintaining a friendship.

But setting the stage in this manner is only the beginning. Studies have shown that it is fairly common for abstinent alcoholics to relapse in the context of a social situation where someone exerts pressure on them to drink (Brownell, Marlatt, Lichtenstein, & Wilson, 1986). This is conceivable, since drinking is a socially accepted way for many individuals to show friendship. People may offer a client a drink simply because they are unaware of the person's drinking problem. At times people know about a client's problem, yet they insist that one drink is not going to hurt. These people typically are not malicious, but simply uninformed regarding the detrimental effects that alcohol has on the client, even in small amounts. Unfortunately, some people are deliberately malevolent and attempt to sabotage the problem drinker by challenging the person to drink.

Sometimes societal pressure takes on a subtle form. For example, if most of Emanuel's friends are heavy drinkers, they may feel uncomfortable around him socially if he is sober. As a result, they gradually stop including him in their get-togethers. Eventually Emanuel is not invited to card games, fishing trips, or to watch ballgames on television. The message is clear: If you do not drink with us, you are no longer welcome in our group. This is another reason why the social and recreational counseling begins early in treatment. It is to be hoped that your clients will be seeking new friends and sources of entertainment. Otherwise they may inadvertently place themselves in high-risk situations by reestablishing relationships with their old drinking companions.

Interestingly, friends are not the only ones who undermine a client's struggle for sobriety. Sometimes the pressure comes from the problem drinker's spouse or partner. This was clearly the case with Henry, who came to the initial counseling session accompanied by his wife, Renee. Henry's drinking had caused him numerous serious problems. And despite three previous unsuccessful attempts to control his drinking, Henry was vehemently opposed to trying disulfiram for a limited period.

When the couple returned for their second appointment, Henry announced that he was now willing to try Antabuse. He had discovered that it was not as easy for him to stay away from alcohol as he had anticipated. To the therapist's surprise, Renee suddenly objected to Henry's decision to take Antabuse. She raised a variety of concerns about possible side effects and health hazards. Finally she stated that she wanted Henry to behave like a "normal" husband who would take her out on Saturday nights for dinner and drinks, and occasionally to dance. She complained that going out would not be much fun if they could not have a couple of drinks to relax them. Needless to say, the therapist pointed out how she was placing her husband in a difficult situation by expecting him to do something that he was not capable of handling this early in treatment. In a later session, Renee's ambivalence about their marital relationship surfaced fully.

The examples above illustrate how subtle or direct pressures from the problem drinker's social environment can make it difficult to maintain sobriety. Consequently, informing friends and family about the decision to stop drinking and enlisting their support is only the first stage of drink-refusal training. Teaching clients actual drink-refusal strategies and having them practice resisting pressure assertively without feeling guilty are important elements that will be detailed shortly.

Reviewing High-Risk Situations

The second phase of drink-refusal training involves reviewing the client's high-risk drinking situations. Start by referring to the individual's Functional Analysis for Drinking Behavior chart. Have your client examine the external triggers for drinking; that is, those environmental factors that often are associated with drinking episodes. In addition, ask your client to generate between five and ten more situations in which a slip seems possible. Often it is helpful for the client to list the ten most frequent places in which he or she drank before entering treatment. But despite these prompts, some clients will claim that they cannot think of any future situations in which they might be tempted to drink. With considerable probing they may still generate only one or two. In these cases a client should be offered suggestions from previous clients. Some CRA therapists record examples on index cards that can be handed to the client. The individual is then instructed to flip through the cards and to pull out any relevant scenarios. These provide the framework for subsequent role-plays. Below are some suggestions of potential high-risk situations that may be listed on index cards for a client's consideration:

1. You and your spouse are having dinner with some friends in a nice restaurant. For starters, the waiter takes orders for before-dinner drinks. Everyone at the table orders an alcoholic beverage.

2. You attend an office Christmas party. Your boss doesn't know about your problem and approaches you with two alcoholic drinks. He extends you a warm greeting and hands you a glass.

3. You are invited to a wedding. At the reception the bride's mother pushes a glass of champagne on you, although you say you don't want to drink. She insists that one glass won't hurt, and that you simply must toast the happy couple.

4. You ride to work with the same group every day. On Fridays they stop at a liquor store for a 12-pack of beer and drink it on the way home. You are seated in the car when a fellow passenger pops a beer and hands it to you. They all know that you have stopped drinking.

5. You had a problem at work, and you feel as if your boss treated you very unfairly. One of your coworkers realizes how angry you are and says, "You look like you could use a drink. It's almost five o'clock. Let's go over to Brock's tavern."

6. You arrive at a party and feel awkward. Everyone seems to be having a good time, but you feel tense and out of place. A friend comes over and tells you that you need to loosen up. She points you toward the kitchen saying, "Go ahead. You'll find the whiskey and wine on the kitchen table, and the beer's in the fridge."

7. An old friend who you haven't seen in several years shows up at your door one night. He is carrying with him a 6-pack to celebrate your reunion. You tell him that you don't drink anymore, but he insists that you have one for old times' sake.

8. Your new boyfriend has invited you to his parents' house for dinner. He is unaware that you are in treatment for a drinking problem. His mother serves wine with dinner, and without asking she fills your glass.

9. You are kissing and caressing your girlfriend. You would like to become sexually intimate with her, but suddenly you become afraid that you will not be able to perform. It has been a long time since you made love sober. She seems to notice that you are nervous and offers you a drink.

These nine scenarios are simply examples of previous clients' reported high-risk situations. Feel free to add to these, or to prompt your clients in an entirely different way. Once a sizable number of high-risk scenes have been identified, it is time to practice declining drinks assertively during role-plays.

Refusing Drinks Assertively

This segment of drink-refusal training draws heavily from the work of Monti, Abrams, Kadden, and Cooney (1989). In our experience the skills are best attained in a step-by-step fashion. Depending on the client and the situation, any or all of the following steps may be used:

1. Saying, "No, thanks."
2. Watching body language.
3. Suggesting alternatives.
4. Changing the subject.
5. Confronting the aggressor.

The first guideline associated with assertive drink refusal is basic in nature but difficult in practice: to teach the client to say no when offered a drink. This usually is most successful if you begin by asking your client to remember some of the negative consequences suffered because of drinking. Then have your client mentally list the positive gains since the drinking stopped. The no should be linked with positive experiences of sobriety.

With strangers or casual acquaintances your client need not give any reasons for not drinking. A simple "No, thanks" should suffice. People refuse drinks all the time, and nonproblem drinkers never feel compelled to give reasons for rejecting a drink. Clients often are surprised to hear this. They feel obligated to explain what they perceive as their own odd behavior; namely, turning down a drink. So some clients feel more comfortable responding, "No, thank you. I don't drink anymore." Any variation of this theme is certainly acceptable, as long as the individual delivers the message in a positive and firm manner.

Refusing alcoholic beverages from close friends and family members is a somewhat different predicament, since these individuals probably will pressure your client for an explanation. Frequently clients respond by offering bogus excuses such as: "Not now. Maybe later"; "Not today. My stomach's bothering me"; or "I'm on medication, so I better not." One danger of giving such excuses is that it invites these family members and friends to offer the client alcohol again in the near future. Eventually most committed clients decide to face the problem head-on and make their decision to abstain public.

The second step of assertive drink-refusal training is teaching your client to be aware of his or her body language. Words and body language should both convey the speaker's firm decision not to drink. If your client begins to sweat, stumbles over words, looks jittery, or has poor eye contact, the aggressor may decide that the decision is not final. A confident, powerful, verbal "No" that is reflected in the client's nonverbal behavior as well can be very convincing.

A third technique for refusing drinks assertively is to suggest alternatives. For example, a client might say, "No, thanks. I don't drink alcohol, but I'd love a good cup of coffee." Make sure that your client has a reasonable list of alternatives and is fluent using them during role-plays. A fourth effective way to refuse a drink is to change the subject to something other than alcohol or drinking. The new subject may be any unrelated topic, such as the weather, mutual friends, or sports.

The dialogue that follows illustrates how a client might incorporate each of the four drink-refusal guidelines presented thus far. Note that there is no "correct" order for delivering the steps; the client simply should use whatever feels comfortable and effective at the time.

THERAPIST: OK, Dale. I'll act as the aggressor and try to get you to drink. Let's set the scene first. I'm your boss. We're at an office party at my house. Picture yourself walking into the kitchen where all the drinks are being served. I'm going to try to get you to drink with me. I want you to refuse my offer by trying some of the strategies we've just gone over.

CLIENT: This might be hard because I can't tell you off since you're my boss. I have to be nice. OK. I'm ready. I'll give it a try.

THERAPIST [playing boss]: I'm glad you could make it to the party, Dale. Have a beer. I bought these special imports just for the party and they're good and cold.

CLIENT: No, thanks. I noticed your deck out back. Did you build it yourself?

THERAPIST [playing boss]: Come on and have a beer and I'll give you a closer look at the deck.

CLIENT: No thanks on the beer, but I would like a cold soda. Say, is that deck made of redwood or is that just the color of the stain?

THERAPIST: Good job, Dale. You really stuck to your guns. You changed the subject, but when I didn't give in you made your intention clear by suggesting a soda instead. Then you went back to the other topic of the deck. And you sounded committed to your decision throughout. Great job.

Note: The client used the first four methods for refusing a drink. He said, "No, thanks," he delivered it with commitment, he suggested a soda instead, and he changed the subject. Clients can use any or all of these steps, depending on their preference and the persistence of the aggressor.

Unfortunately these first four methods may not discourage some individuals who are offering alcohol to your client. In these cases it may be necessary for your client to take a stronger stand. Confronting the aggressor should be done as a last resort. Typically the confrontation involves the client asking the aggressor why it is so important to get the client to drink; for example:

1. "I've now told you several times that I am not drinking any alcohol, but you keep pushing me to drink. I don't understand. Why is it so important to you that I drink?"
2. "I don't want any alcohol. I'm not sure what it is about that statement that isn't clear. Why do you keep asking me?"

The client should not have to justify his or her actions. By confronting the aggressor, the client turns the tables on the motive of the other person. In most cases this will effectively stop the "pusher." But the client should be prepared for counterattacks and even the temporary loss of a friend.

There are many options regarding assertive ways to decline a drink. But even when clients find several with which they feel comfortable and confident, they harbor some guilt about refusing an alcoholic beverage. They see themselves as inadequate for not being able to drink like a "normal" person. It is also difficult for them because they think they are hurting their friends' feelings, or letting them down. These feelings subside once the clients understand that it is their right not to drink. The longer they are sober and receiving positive reinforcers in new areas of their lives, the easier it is for the guilt to dissipate.

Restructuring Negative Thoughts

The final component of drink-refusal training is a cognitive procedure that examines clients' faulty thought patterns. In essence, this procedure teaches clients to say no to themselves when the temptation to drink presents itself.

Refer again to the client's CRA Functional Analysis for Drinking Behavior chart (see Chapter 2, Appendix 2.A), but this time focus on your client's internal triggers. As you recall, these are the thoughts and feelings that lead to drinking. Cognitive restructuring entails having your client challenge each thought that has become associated with drinking behaviors. The evidence for the thought should be examined, and a positive thought not associated with drinking should be substituted instead. Sometimes a double-column exercise is useful. Have your client record the self-defeating statement in one column, and a positive counter statement in the opposite column. Then discuss with your client how realistic each statement is. Illustrate how to replace the old, negative, drinking-associated thought with a new positive one. Have your client repeat the new thought several times. While practicing this thought substitution, the client should try to imagine the new feelings that automatically would accompany these positive thoughts. A brief demonstration of the technique follows.

THERAPIST: Barbara, one of the thoughts you listed on your chart as a drinking trigger was, "I've had an awful day. I just need a drink to relax." I think you can see now how you're setting yourself up to drink. Do you really *need* a drink to relax? Can you think of something else you might say to yourself when you're feeling awful and like you need a drink to relax?

CLIENT: Well, I guess I could say, "What an awful day! Maybe I should treat myself to some ice cream tonight."

THERAPIST: That's a good start. You're challenging the thought of needing a drink to relax. And if you ended up having ice cream instead, how do you think you'd feel?

CLIENT: Probably pretty good afterwards. Maybe not as good at first, but at the end of the evening I'd feel better about myself.

THERAPIST: I bet you could come up with a number of nondrinking behaviors that helped you relax. But let's look again at your actual thoughts when you first start thinking about drinking as an option. Can you come up with something nice and supportive to say to yourself when you've had a bad day; something that will make you feel better right then and there?

Note: The therapist looks now for intangible "rewards", such as positive thoughts that lead to good feelings about oneself. This type of reinforcer is immediate and potentially more generalizable.

CLIENT: Sure. Hmmm. I could say, "I don't need alcohol to feel better. I've been doing really well without it, so there's no reason to spoil things. So I've had a bad day; big deal. I already know about two good things that are going to happen tomorrow."

THERAPIST: That was a whole string of nice comments and good reasons why you don't need alcohol. As you picture yourself saying those things, how do you think you'd feel?

CLIENT: A lot better, I'd imagine.

Cognitive restructuring generally takes a fair amount of practice. Help your client challenge several negative drinking-related thoughts during the session so that he or she will be better prepared to attempt it in the upcoming week. Remind your client to pay close attention to the feelings that result from the new positive thoughts. Review the outcome in the next session.

◆ ◆

This chapter has presented three major types of skills training programs: communication skills, problem solving, and drink refusal. Most alcohol-abusing clients require some combination of these skills programs. This should be apparent upon reviewing an individual's treatment plan. Be sure to list the specific skills training program in the "Intervention" section of the client's Goals of Counseling form, and indicate the allotted training period. Additional skills-building techniques suitable for inclusion in the "Intervention" section will be introduced in the next chapter.

Appendix 6.A *SIMULATED BLACKBOARD PRESENTATION OF PROBLEM-SOLVING APPROACH*

Define Problem

- Can't fall asleep
- Mind races
- Can't seem to relax

Related Problems

- Caffeine (Coke, coffee)
- Nicotine (cigarettes)
- Sits in front of TV all evening

Brainstorming

- Sleepytime tea
- Go for a walk
- Cut down smoking at night
- Cut down coffee at night
- Hot bath before bed
- Read a book
- Relaxation tape
- Meditate
- Drink
- Take Valium
- Quiet music

Solutions

- Sleepytime tea (5 times per week)
- No coffee after dinner (5 times per week)
- Eight cigarettes after dinner (5 times per week)

7

Additional CRA
Techniques

The Community Reinforcement Approach aspires to replace in a timely manner a client's old maladaptive drinking behaviors with new appropriate coping strategies. This chapter reviews a number of the techniques utilized by CRA therapists to accomplish that goal. Frequently these techniques are used in conjunction with some of the procedures outlined already, such as problem solving and communication skills training. CRA therapists believe, however, that the most sophisticated techniques and coping strategies will fall short if an alcohol-abusing client does not have a job.

JOB COUNSELING

Purpose

Satisfying employment and financial security are extremely important aspects of daily living. A good job potentially provides many valuable sources of reinforcement: enhanced self-esteem, stimulating challenges, praise from supervisors, pleasant social interactions with coworkers, and financial rewards (basic salary and raises). Obviously money also opens the door to a host of other material reinforcers, such as a home, car, and entertainment. Yet another advantage of steady employment is that it serves as a deterrent to excessive drinking and drug use, because of the structure it introduces into the day. In summary, there are numerous reasons why alcohol-abusing clients, in particular, benefit from having a job.

General Description

CRA's job counseling program utilizes a disciplined step-by-step approach to assist clients in obtaining and keeping satisfying employment. Training is based largely on Azrin and Besalel's *Job Club Counselor's Manual* (1980). This book carefully describes each procedure and supplies excellent worksheets that can be modified to fit the needs of any client or program. The premise underlying this approach is that finding a job is a full-time job.

The *Job Club Counselor's Manual* was designed to be used in a club or group format. Unfortunately, most treatment programs today have neither the equivalent of a Job Finding Club nor the resources to run a full-time job-finding program. Therefore it is imperative that all therapists be familiar with fundamental job-seeking procedures. The guidelines that follow have been adapted so that they may be delivered on a one-to-one basis.

Developing a Résumé

Developing a solid résumé is an important first step in the job-finding process. The real purpose of a résumé is to create a sufficiently favorable impression such that the applicant is granted an interview. With this in mind, a résumé should not show large gaps between jobs, even if the client was temporarily unemployed because of drinking or drug use. These gaps should be described instead as periods of self-employment, or as times when the client was rethinking career goals. If an interview is secured, the nature of these difficult times and the resolution of the problem can be explained more fully.

In order to determine which information should be included in a résumé, discuss with your client all prior jobs and training. Oftentimes clients inadvertently overlook certain skills, or they elect not to mention ones that they consider trivial. So encourage your client to describe former job duties in great detail, and develop a list of *all* the skills involved. Remind your client that positive personal qualities, such as patience, loyalty, or perseverance, should be mentioned on a résumé as well. One exercise that helps highlight these personal characteristics is having the client role-play the comments a coworker might offer about him or her.

The résumé should be carefully typed, and an introductory cover letter should be developed to accompany it. Forms useful for the construction of each are located in the *Job Club Counselor's Manual* (Azrin & Besalel, 1980). Additionally, there are several computer software programs available today that assist in the writing of résumés.

Avoiding Jobs with High Relapse Potential

At this point you will have a clear idea of the types of jobs your client has held in the past. If the topic has not already been explored, be sure to discuss the relapse potential associated with each of these positions. Your objective is to steer clients away from future jobs that are high-risk situations. Their functional analysis charts should be informative here. Frequently it becomes apparent that clients can make considerably more money at a certain familiar job, but the particular position has a historical association with drinking. Nonetheless, clients often express an interest in pursuing this type of work when they begin their job search. They feel confident about being able to secure employment in that field again. The thought of switching fields may be overwhelming at first, but it often is the only reasonable plan for maintaining sobriety.

Completing Job Applications

Clients next should be taught the skills necessary to fill out a job application appropriately. One component of this task involves showing clients how to diplomatically address difficult questions, so that they are still presenting themselves in a favorable light. At times this may entail leaving a question blank. For example, suppose a question pointedly asks whether an individual has a drug or alcohol problem. It would be advisable to skip such a potentially damaging question so that the topic could be discussed in person with the employer. This would enable the client to explain that treatment is ongoing, and that the problem is under control. If the client answered yes to the question outright, in all probability the employer would not invite the person for an interview. The opportunity to describe one's current success in that area would be lost.

If possible, collect job applications from a variety of employers in the community so that clients can practice answering all types of questions while receiving feedback. Be prepared to review the basics as well, such as the need either to use a typewriter or to print neatly and legibly. Too often an application is set aside simply because the employer has to struggle to read it. Furthermore, the care with which an application is completed creates an initial impression about the applicant.

Generating Job Leads

Once the client has a good résumé and is proficient at completing job applications, the next step is to generate job leads. The recommended approach is a structured procedure that entails first listing a series of job leads, and then documenting all relevant information pertaining to contacts. It is fairly common for clients to be reluctant to adhere to this planned method, however. Instead many prefer to "hit the streets," responding impulsively to whatever is available at that point in time. There are two problems with such a strategy: (1) It does not allow time to prepare for the interview, and (2) there is no opportunity to discuss the appropriateness of the position in terms of the client's treatment plan and the relapse potential.

Generating job leads can be done several ways. Since most jobs are secured through word of mouth, one way to obtain leads is to ask family and friends if they know of any employment possibilities. Other leads may come from former employers and co-workers. Additionally, your client may rely on the yellow pages of the phone book. If so, be sure the client not only checks the main listing for a job but also explores listings for related fields. For example, suppose your client is seeking employment as a salesperson in a lumber yard. Have him or her look in the yellow pages under lumber yards, as well as lumber distributors, lumber mills, and lumber treating. This will widen the range of possible jobs in a specific area of interest. Your client should then list all possible places for employment on a job leads form. This form should include the name of the company, the date the company was called, the name of the person in charge of hiring, the telephone number, the address, and the result of the call. The log should also contain categories for second and third calls, so that follow-up phone calls are an automatic part of the process. In addition to the yellow pages, newspaper want ads and job postings at employment agencies can be useful in generating job leads. A minimum of ten job leads should be identified before the client begins to make any phone calls of inquiry.

Telephone Skills Training

The job seeker should rely on the telephone to arrange interviews, since writing individual letters or visiting each job site in person is time consuming and costly. But prior to placing any calls, clients should be trained to communicate in a concise and positive manner on the telephone. The following format is suggested:

1. Introduce yourself.
2. Ask for the name of the department head, or the person responsible for hiring.
3. Address that individual by name and introduce yourself.
4. Give your qualifications briefly.
5. Request an interview.
6. If an interview is not granted for a current position, inquire about an interview in the event that an opening occurs later.
7. If this request is denied as well, ask for other job leads in the area.
8. Ask permission to use this individual's name for job leads.
9. Inquire about a reasonable time to call back about future job openings.

Role-play all nine steps until the client has mastered phone procedures for securing job interviews.

Interview Rehearsal

Assume your client has the first real interview arranged. Assist in the preparation by discussing the importance of punctuality, proper dress, and personal hygiene. Be sure that transportation has been arranged as well. Then focus specifically on improving your client's interviewing skills through behavioral rehearsal. The *Job Club Counselor's Manual* provides many excellent examples of typical interview questions and appropriate responses (Azrin & Besalel, 1980, Appendix 42). Practice a series of these role-plays, such that they become progressively more challenging. In this manner your client will be able to handle a wide variety of questions that may be posed by prospective employers. And since building the client's confidence is one of the most important outcomes of this procedure, use positive reinforcement whenever possible.

Job finding can be difficult and very frustrating. Your clients must be prepared to be rejected during the process. Planning for this probable event will help prevent them from becoming too discouraged and losing their motivation. Clients need to understand that *not* getting a job is just part of job finding. Remind them that this is one more example of a problem in need of a solution.

Learning How to Keep a Job

Many people in treatment for alcohol problems have more trouble keeping a job than finding one. Consequently the process does not end once your client has obtained a position. Instead you should begin to explore the nature of past work difficulties. One helpful exercise is to have your client list the problems that have been associated with work in the past, and any foreseeable ones for the new job.

Next discuss the warning signals or precursors of these problems. For example, be sure to examine relationships with supervisors and other employees. Determine whether drinking on the job, tardiness, or abuse of sick time were factors associated with job termination. Did emotional problems or preoccupation with alcohol play a role in the loss of a job? In essence, pinpoint internal and external "triggers" that led to job-related trouble.

Once all possible problems and their precursors have been listed, use the problem-solving intervention demonstrated in Chapter 6 to seek positive solutions. Then place all potential solutions in a column opposite the problem descriptions. Obtain a firm commitment from your client to try several solutions. Proceed with role-plays if any of the problems involve communication difficulties. Be prepared to check weekly with your client about both positive and negative job developments.

The remaining sections of this chapter introduce five additional CRA procedures that are available to supplement the basic behavioral skills training.

SOLUTION ORIENTATION

It is not at all unusual for therapists from many different theoretical orientations to begin sessions with a general question such as, "How are things going?" or "Where would you like to begin today?" In the interest of efficiency and based on past success, the CRA therapist generally avoids such open statements. The therapist is determined to move quickly to a discussion of solutions for specific, relevant problems. Opening statements often pertain to defined goals and homework assignments. For example, a therapist might ask, "Did you have an opportunity to try the new Social Club?" or, "Have you practiced your drink-refusal skills since I saw you last?" Session time is spent on tasks, such as explaining or practicing new procedures, or ascertaining why the client did not properly implement the old procedures. The ultimate goal is to provide the client with problem-solving strategies that later may be utilized for a wide variety of difficulties. In essence, the entire therapy process is solution oriented rather than problem oriented, but not at the expense of sacrificing empathy.

The dialogue that follows is an example of the therapist moving the client from a problem orientation to a *Solution Orientation* at the start of a session. Note the points the therapist has been trained to cover:

1. Inquire about homework assignments or any other progress toward treatment goals.
2. Make certain that the client understands the reasons for any change; whether it is a success or a failure.
3. Reinforce the client's efforts.
4. Express appropriate empathy.
5. Move forward toward a solution of a new problem instead of dwelling on a description of the problem itself.
6. Look for similar problems in the client's recent past to determine which solutions were previously effective.
7. Use problem solving or another relevant procedure to address any remaining issues.

THERAPIST: Ann, what progress have you made on your treatment goals during this last week?

CLIENT: Well, I did stay sober. But I'll tell you, my boss is really giving me a hard time. He picks on me constantly. Everybody else gets away with murder, and they don't work half as hard as me. But if I do anything slightly wrong, he climbs all over me.

THERAPIST: OK. I'll talk to you about your boss in a minute. But first of all, congratulations on staying sober again. That's a big accomplishment; let's not downplay it! What do you think helped you the most with your goal of staying sober this week?

CLIENT: I don't know. It wasn't as hard this week. John really seemed to be on my side. I wonder if those marital sessions that we just started had something to do with it.

THERAPIST: You're probably right. Your husband can see how hard you're trying, and you're learning how to communicate with each other better. Sounds like a good reason to keep working away in those sessions.

Note: Since the new problem did not appear to be a crisis, the therapist decided to review progress first. She reinforced the client's achievement, and then made certain that Ann knew *why* it was easier to stay sober this past week. In the event of a crisis, this review could have been saved until later in the session.

THERAPIST: Now, how about if we do some problem solving around this issue with your boss? It sounds like he's really got you feeling frustrated.

CLIENT: I just can't stand him. He's such a knothead. He probably only got the job because he's related to the owner.

THERAPIST: Ann, you're obviously very upset, and probably for good reason. But let's see if we can move forward and focus instead on how to solve this problem. We certainly can't change your boss. But if you do some problem solving you may find a better way to deal with him. Maybe we can get some ideas by reviewing how you successfully handled your brother when you felt like he was always giving you a hard time.

CLIENT: OK. I understand. But my boss is still a jerk.

Although the therapist certainly wanted to acknowledge Ann's feelings, she did not want to encourage her to spend an excessive amount of time in unproductive complaining. This is not to say that Ann's concerns were unjustified; only that the goal was to move the client forward in a direction that could solve the problem instead of dwelling upon it. The therapist began by reminding the client that she had solved a similar problem with her brother. This successful solution would be reviewed, and if possible, applied to the current problem. The therapist would rely on the actual problem-solving strategy, whether modifying the previous solution or generating an entirely new one.

PROMPT RULE

Periodically you will encounter clients who initially are unwilling or unable to participate in the establishment of their treatment goals. These clients simply may be nonresponsive, or they may state that they are uncertain as to what they wish to gain from treatment. The *Prompt Rule* is a mechanism for encouraging a nonresponsive or indecisive client to engage in the process of formulating some specific therapy goals.

An illustration using the prompt rule with a resistant client follows. The therapist first attempts to elicit any kind of response, using a forced-choice question format. This is then shaped into a more informative answer. You should note that typically a therapist would not provide the degree of structure shown in this example. This format should be reserved for extreme cases.

THERAPIST: OK, Joan, so you noted on your Goals of Counseling form that you want to improve your social life by adding new non-alcohol-related activities. What kind of activities did you have in mind?

CLIENT: [*Long pause*] I don't know.

THERAPIST: You seem to be having trouble coming up with some choices. Would you like some help?

CLIENT: I don't care.

Note: At this point you should suggest something specific in an effort to simply engage the client in the process.

THERAPIST: I remember seeing on your functional analysis chart that you enjoyed gardening on weekends. Do you have any interest in finding a way to make it a more sociable activity?

CLIENT: I don't know. I'm not sure I want to.

Note: It often is useful at this stage to resort to a multiple-choice format.

THERAPIST: Sometimes it's hard to get started, isn't it? Let me go ahead and give you a number of options. Which of the following sounds worth pursuing: finding a way to make gardening a social event, joining a hiking group, taking a pottery class, or swimming at a public pool?

CLIENT: I'm not sure.

Note: If the client still is having difficulty, break down the choices by comparing two options at a time.

THERAPIST: Well, how about you choose the better of two alternatives? If you had to pick one, which would you prefer, Joan, adding gardening or hiking as a new social activity?

CLIENT: I'm not sure how you'd make gardening a social event.

Note: The client is giving some indication of interest in this one activity. If the therapist decides to pursue it as a realistic option, problem solving could be conducted to work out the details.

The Prompt Rule helps the client accept responsibility for treatment, which in turn often serves to motivate him or her. If after several attempts with the Prompt Rule a client still is totally unwilling to participate in the treatment process, you may decide to probe the resistance directly, or to resort to Motivation Reversal as a final option (p. 131). As noted earlier, the Prompt Rule is a technique that typically is not advocated by most therapy approaches, since it forces choices instead of allowing the client to generate them. Again, CRA resorts to this format only in extreme cases, and it does so in the interest of moving the therapy process along in a timely fashion.

DURATION TRAINING

Convincing clients to refrain from going back to their old drinking "hangouts" is difficult, yet necessary in most cases. The external triggers for drinking in these environments are just too powerful. Nevertheless, even the most motivated client occasionally will find him- or herself in a familiar drinking environment. One known contributor to patterns of excessive drinking involves the client choosing to remain in this high-risk environment for an extended period of time. Consequently it seems logical to reduce the time interval in which the problem drinker is exposed to alcohol consumption cues. The *Duration Training* procedure is designed specifically to decrease the amount of time engaged in alcohol-related activities and environments.

Begin by determining the client's most common setting for drinking behavior outside the home, such as a bar or a friend's house. Then, ask him or her to estimate how much time usually is spent in this place. Next, see if the client is willing to decrease the amount of time there, and if so, by how much. Ideally the activity will be eliminated altogether, but some clients elect to try limiting it. Given the latter scenario, Duration Training next entails having the client imagine that he or she is in that typical drinking location, and that it is a reasonable time to leave. The client actually should practice announcing the intention to go, and review the benefits of doing so. It is often worthwhile to include an in vivo training phase as well. If possible, it should be conducted when the client is taking disulfiram and is in the presence of social support. This will reduce the probability of a failure experience and increase the likelihood of social reinforcement for successful completion of these activities.

The second part of this training sequence involves decreasing the amount of time spent in other environments that also involve a drinking component, but which have many positive, nondrinking aspects to them as well. These environments may include certain sports, family outings, and other structured events where alcohol is not the main focus but nevertheless is present. If possible, you again would want the client to replace these activities with new, productive ones that do not involve alcohol. But this is unrealistic in many cases, and, consequently, you should assist the client in finding ways to decrease the amount of time spent in these activities.

The next dialogue illustrates how to reduce the duration of exposure to alcohol cues while attending a high-risk event. The critical component is having a well-developed plan in place prior to attending the activity.

THERAPIST: Mary Lou, you mentioned earlier that you were going to have supper at your in-laws on Sunday. Isn't that one of the high-risk activities for your drinking?

CLIENT: Yes, but what can I do? It's my mother-in-law's birthday. If I don't go I'll create even more trouble.

THERAPIST: Is there any way to reduce the time you will be there, so that you won't be tempted to drink for such a long period? Remember our problem-solving procedure? Can you find a good solution?

CLIENT: I've been thinking about my options. I probably could leave early, right after dinner. That way I'd avoid most of the drinking.

THERAPIST: And how exactly would you do that? What would you say?

CLIENT: I could either say I wasn't feeling well, or just tell them that I had things planned; that I was sorry, but I needed to go.

THERAPIST: They both sound reasonable. Which one would you like to try?

CLIENT: I guess I'll just say I have things that I need to do. I'd feel more comfortable saying that than making up excuses about being sick.

THERAPIST: Good. Now what's going to get in the way of you actually leaving right after dinner as planned?

CLIENT: Nothing, now that I've made up my mind. I've done it before and it works OK as long as Bruce stays there with the kids for a little while longer.

The client generated and then adopted a reasonable plan for reducing exposure to alcohol cues in an unavoidable high-risk social event. The therapist merely checked to determine how carefully she had thought through the particulars of her plan, including the consequences. In this case Mary Lou knew that most of the drinking would happen after the meal. She planned on spending as little time as possible in such a risky situation. She knew exactly what to avoid and how to do it. The therapist would inquire about the outcome at the next session, and would assist in modifying the plan for future encounters if necessary.

MOTIVATION REVERSAL

Motivation Reversal is a technique that is quite similar to paradoxical intention. Within CRA it is used to deal with clients who have been only minimally compliant and who seem to generate innumerable excuses for their lack of progress. This procedure involves discontinuing all direct, obvious efforts to motivate the client. Instead it subtly places the responsibility for change entirely on the client and, in some cases, the Concerned Other. Interesting shifts in motivation often follow.

Consider, for example, a case in which a new client's wife reports that she has not been administering her husband's disulfiram. Also, the couple states that they have only been attending sessions biweekly because they felt that weekly appointments were unnecessary. Using Motivation Reversal you first would convey a message that on the surface applauds their private decision to modify their treatment plan. You would emphasize the positive changes that the husband has made, and state that the wife probably really knows what is best for him, since they have so much contact with each other. A review of some of the couple's past problems would follow, with you then discussing how to handle those problems on their own *when* they arise in the future. As you begin to minimize the extent of your involvement in the therapy, typically the couple would show signs of apprehension at the notion of losing your guidance and support. They would realize that they are not yet ready to tackle the problems completely on their own, and would resist the notion of you "abandoning" them. At this point you would introduce some basic requirements for continued therapy.

It is important to remember that to be effective this procedure requires that the therapist have a thorough understanding of a client's problems, and that they have a reasonable relationship. The former concern will be satisfied if a comprehensive functional analysis has been conducted.

A second example of Motivation Reversal follows. It is a dialogue between a therapist and a court-referred client who is resistant to any kind of significant behavior change. The important elements of the technique are noted as they occur in the conversation, and are then outlined at its conclusion.

THERAPIST: Hi, Nick, how are you doing today?

CLIENT: I'm doing pretty good.

THERAPIST: I'm surprised to hear you say that. We've been working on issues for about five weeks, and it seems like there aren't a lot of changes going on.

CLIENT: Well, I'm coming to therapy. I mean, I'm doing everything that the probation officer said I have to do. He said I have to come here, so I'm coming.

THERAPIST: Your probation officer told me you haven't followed through with other recommendations, such as getting a job. You haven't even looked for one seriously. This is a requirement of your probation. Let me remind you that we are talking five or six years in jail. And I'm still waiting for you to bring Laurie in.

Note: Here the therapist gently confronts the client for his failure to look for a job and to bring his wife to a session. He reminds the client of the probable consequences; namely, going to jail.

CLIENT: I don't want to go back to the joint, but at the same time I feel like I only have to come down here. So I am.

THERAPIST: You haven't done the homework assignments either. So all you are doing is coming to therapy. You are marking time. And I feel that at this juncture in your therapy this isn't productive. Quite honestly, I can't see where we are going. You're still hanging around with the same crowd. You're still going to bars.

CLIENT: I'm not drinking, though.

THERAPIST: No, and I'm glad to hear that. I'm worried about how long it's going to last, though. Nick, this may sound odd at first, but to be honest, I am so concerned about you that I think it would be best for us to discontinue therapy.

CLIENT: What . . . what do you mean?

THERAPIST: Well, I just think that we've come to a point where therapy is not being productive. I'm uncomfortable with you just doing your own thing. I'll write a letter to your probation officer and let him know that we don't seem to be a good team, that we're not making sufficient progress. But I bet the two of you can figure something out. Another form of therapy might better suit your needs, get you on track. We're just not making it. I'm sure you'll be able to find a therapist who is comfortable with you setting up your own program, and being real independent.

CLIENT: Well, I don't know if I want to do that because they told me to come down here for this program, and I don't want to go to AA meetings.

THERAPIST: Nick, I don't want to keep pushing you. Maybe this isn't even the right time for you to make these changes. Originally you agreed to get a job, to look for new friends, and to bring Laurie in. But you're not doing any of these things. Maybe you're right; maybe these things aren't important now. But I'm worried about you having a relapse because you haven't made certain basic changes. So what I need to do is call your probation officer and let him know our status. Just sit down with him and decide on another program and another therapist. Ethically I can't keep working with you if I don't see that I'm helping.

Note: The therapist resorted to Motivation Reversal here. Notice that he did not simply blame the client for the lack of progress. Instead he accepted partial responsibility by stating that they did not work well together. He remained optimistic about the client being able to find a new therapist who would be a better match with the client's "independent" style. At this point the responsibility for treatment was shifted back to the client.

CLIENT: Well, I don't know if I want to find another program. I feel comfortable here. I've been coming now for more than a month. Why do you think I need to go someplace else? And you don't need to call my probation officer.

THERAPIST: But we're getting nowhere, Nick. Nowhere.

CLIENT: I just started. And I'm not even drinking!

Note: This is a common reaction to the Motivation Reversal procedure. The client realizes that all responsibility for his treatment is being handed over to him. Although he enjoys his "freedom," he is not ready to accept the consequences.

THERAPIST: But Nick, you know what I require. Why don't you tell me what you are willing to do right now to stay in therapy with me. How about finding a job?

Note: The therapist realizes that there is room to bargain at this point. He decides to pursue the matter by getting the client to agree to some minimal commitments.

CLIENT: Well, . . . if, . . . uh, . . . I've been looking.

THERAPIST: You've turned down a lot of jobs simply because you didn't think they paid enough. We talked about the importance of having work. And it is part of your probation. You refused to go through the Job Finding Program. You said that you would do it on your own. Would you be willing to get involved in the Job Finding Program, starting tomorrow? Would you do that?

CLIENT: Well, yeah, I could do that. I suppose I should.

THERAPIST: OK. And are you willing to set up a therapy appointment with Laurie for this week?

CLIENT: I guess. If I have to.

THERAPIST: No guess. This is your decision.

CLIENT: Well, does this mean that I can just keep coming to this program?

THERAPIST: Yes. If you show these commitments, I'll reassess my situation with you. I would like to work with you. But I don't want to be used as someone who just marks time with you and sends reports saying you're coming. Because in reality, if you don't stay sober and out of trouble, you're going to end up going back to jail. And I don't want to see that happen to you, or your wife.

CLIENT: All right, I'm willing to do more.

Note: Once it was apparent that the client did not want to find a new therapist, the counselor introduced some requirements of his own for the client to continue in therapy. Setting up contingencies was one way to increase the client's motivation.

Although confrontation of this type is not a common feature of CRA, occasionally it is used. You should note a few unique aspects of the CRA type of confrontation:

1. The confrontation was executed in a nonderogatory, nonblaming manner. It focused on the types of behavior that the individual did or did not perform, as opposed to criticizing the person per se.
2. It tied in the client's main motivator: avoiding jail.
3. It was directed toward getting the client to comply with the requirements of the program; namely, obtaining a job and starting marital therapy.
4. The confrontation did not entail threatening that the therapist would in any way be instrumental in revoking the probation.
5. The therapist accepted partial responsibility in stating that he did not think they were working well together as a team.
6. The therapist used a positive reframe for the client's resistance by referring to it as the client's "independent" style.
7. The responsibility for treatment was shifted back to the client.
8. A contingency was introduced, in which the client could remain with this therapist if he followed through with certain treatment requirements.

It is important to use this technique only when you have established a solid rapport with a client, and you truly understand the person's reinforcers. The technique will not be successful if the client receives no rewards for remaining in therapy. Also, it is crucial to intervene at a time when clients have to make a choice. Most often they choose the line of least resistance and return to their current therapy, as opposed to finding a new program or beginning with a new individual therapist.

One of the guiding principles of Motivation Reversal is that it should not be utilized unless one is quite certain that the client will choose to remain in therapy. Regardless, you should always consider the possibility that the client may decide to leave. You would not want the individual to be set up for inevitable failure. So in the event that the client terminates, make every effort to refer him or her to another program.

INDEPENDENCE TRAINING

One of the goals of CRA is to teach basic skills to the client or couple so that they can resolve their own problems in the future. *Independence Training* is a strategy for preparing clients to incorporate these skills into their daily lives. It is composed primarily of behavioral rehearsal and feedback during sessions, and homework assignments throughout the week. Clients come to understand that they can troubleshoot most of their problems, but in the event that they require assistance, they always can return to therapy, detox, disulfiram, or Job Finding.

Independence Training appears in many forms. Relatively early in therapy it may involve having the therapist leave the room temporarily while a couple attempts to problem solve on their own. The therapist would check on progress upon returning, and then supply feedback and positive reinforcement. Setting up and testing an Early Warning System (see Chapter 10: CRA Relapse Prevention) is part of Independence Training as well. This procedure enables couples to identify drinking triggers, and to avoid a potential relapse on their own through problem solving. Establishing a social and recreational plan that is alcohol free is another component. Ideally the client will see others as role models for nondrinking behavior, and eventually will become more integrated into a nondrinking society. Yet one more aspect of Independence Training is being certain that couples or individuals get linked to the appropriate support groups, such as AA or Al-Anon.

In the latter stages of therapy, Independence Training involves an actual weaning process, whereby sessions become spaced further and further apart. It is common to move from weekly to biweekly, and then monthly sessions. Often clients become apprehensive at this time, and symptoms escalate in response. One way to deal with this reaction is to adopt an open door policy. Essentially the therapist is available on the phone to assist them in the transition, primarily through problem solving of minor difficulties. Furthermore, follow-up sessions are scheduled every 2 to 3 months.

The last stage of Independence Training is the termination session. An outline of the points to cover in this final therapy session is presented below:

1. Review the client's progress. Briefly cover the presenting problems and their current status.
2. Discuss what you and the client each view as the most beneficial aspect of the treatment in addressing these problems.
3. Check to see that the client fully understands how to carry out the relevant procedures.
4. Reinforce the client's efforts and hard work.
5. Discuss any unmet goals on the Goals of Counseling form, and plans for achieving them.
6. Check to ensure that the client has a healthy nondrinking support system established.

7. Discuss any concerns the client might have about proceeding alone.
8. Remind the client about the open door policy, in which phone calls are always an option and booster sessions are welcomed.
9. Schedule a definite follow-up appointment to take place within 2 to 3 months.
10. Inform the client that you will call at least once a month prior to the follow-up appointment. This demonstration of support also serves to increase the probability that the client will call you if a problem arises, and will attend the follow-up appointment.

♦   ♦

This chapter has presented a variety of useful procedures for helping a client establish a rewarding, nondrinking lifestyle. At the top of the list were instructions for finding and keeping a job. It is assumed that these procedures will only supplement the basic strategies: communication skills, problem-solving skills and drink-refusal training. The next chapter focuses specifically on methods for enhancing an individual's new sober social life.

8

Social and Recreational Counseling*

One extremely important component of CRA treatment is assisting the client in developing satisfying social and recreational activities that compete with alcohol use and support sobriety. When clients first seek treatment they often are totally enmeshed in a "drinking culture" in which friendships and recreational activities center around drinking. In essence, drinking is a prerequisite for maintaining these social relationships. Moreover, it is not unusual for clients to find themselves ostracized from former friends when they stop drinking. Given the powerful influence peer group affiliations and social interactions have on drinking behavior, either circumstance readily can serve as a trigger point for relapse. Changing peer reference groups and developing healthier alcohol-free social outlets are exceedingly difficult and require training during the early phase of the CRA counseling process.

Developing a Healthy Social Life

Begin the topic with a discussion of the importance of developing healthy social and recreational activities. To illustrate the relationship

---

*This chapter was written with John H. Mallams.

between drinking and social activities and affiliations, ask the client to identify friends and activities that have always been associated with the use of alcohol. Commonly these activities include going to bars or pool halls, playing cards, eating at certain restaurants, or just "hanging around" with former drinking buddies. Next, ask the client to identify individuals and social situations which usually are not associated with drinking. These may include family outings, church activities, AA meetings, movies, hobbies, and some sporting events. Once the client demonstrates a sufficient understanding of the relationship between his or her drinking and social life, encourage the client to make a commitment to establish new friendships and "try out" alternative social activities supportive of sobriety.

Identifying Areas of Interest

Your next task is to pinpoint the client's areas of interest. During this process be careful not to force your own bias regarding recreational activities on the client; instead, identify activities that truly are reinforcing for him or her. Perhaps one of the most difficult parts of this process is finding a new activity that the client is even willing to try. You also should be aware of the importance of selecting social events that can be scheduled during "high-risk" drinking periods; namely, at times when the client is most likely to use alcohol.

Periodically a client appears unable to identify a desirable nondrinking recreational activity. One proven technique for generating ideas is to ask the person to "Name three people whom you really admire. What do these individuals do for recreation?" In the likely event that the client does not know the answer to this, an assignment is made to find out. Regardless of whether the client named television or sports personalities, or family members or friends, this simple task usually results in a list of potentially enjoyable social activities.

Another useful technique is to have the client simply write down five to ten recreational activities. Ask the client to agree to experiment with one for a week. The attitude conveyed is, "Try it, you might like it." This procedure will be discussed further in the next section, Reinforcer Sampling.

Frequently it is worthwhile to discuss accessible local activities such as movies, plays, concerts, and adult sport leagues. These events should be ones in which alcohol is not a major element, and where clients can meet new nondrinking friends. Church groups, civic organizations, and local self-help groups are other sources of nondrinking activities that will give the client quality social and recreational experiences and will, at the same time, support sobriety.

During this entire process it will be necessary to remind the client that the ultimate goal is to establish and maintain satisfying relationships with Concerned Others who will support the client's abstinence. With this objective in mind, the client should be encouraged to start, if possible, with an activity that involves someone who is already supportive of his or her sobriety. The client should inform this individual and other friends about this goal of remaining abstinent, and the need for their support. If the client does not have an existing support system and lacks the skills to obtain one, then communication skills training will need to be emphasized early in treatment (see Chapter 6).

Community Access

A major focus of CRA is to assist the client in establishing alternative social interactions and recreational activities that discourage drinking and reward sobriety. While many regularly occurring activities already available within the local community certainly would be appropriate choices, clients frequently profess a basic lack of information about where to even look for such people and events. *Community Access* is the process whereby you provide your client with a variety of reasonable, accessible options. In order to do this, it is critical for you to be knowledgeable about suitable community resources. This extends beyond having a basic community resource manual. In addition, your resource guide should include descriptive information about the suitability of each activity in terms of meeting an individual client's unique needs. For example, the various local AA groups could be rated on a continuum of supportive to confrontational style. Those that accept the use of psychotropic medications could be noted as well. The bottom line is that an uninformed recommendation from you might result in a negative experience for a client. The final outcome could be diminished trust in you and future noncompliance.

Reinforcer Sampling

Identifying suitable areas of interest is only the beginning. Many clients are reluctant to follow through and actually participate in a novel activity, especially when they are sober. The process of "trying out" or experimenting with alternative activities is called *Reinforcer Sampling*. Clients need to sample activities in order to determine if there is any potential for enjoyment. Further, the more one samples, the more likely it is that one will find rewarding events.

Explore the basis for a client's reluctance to become involved in a new social network. Discuss any apprehension about being accepted by strangers, and offer solid suggestions regarding activities with a low risk for rejection. For instance, the client might be encouraged to take a class in an identified interest at a local community college. If a client enjoys photography, for example, he or she could be asked to enroll in a photography course. Explain that the client already has much in common with the rest of the class: an interest in photography. Consequently this will provide an initial topic of conversation. This also will help the client use the newly acquired communication skills in a nonthreatening, sober environment.

Given the fact that it may be difficult to encourage a client to attend new activities, you should proceed slowly and hold reasonable expectations. Since participating in a new activity becomes easier with practice, advise your clients to routinely schedule recreational events. Many individuals find that they are more apt to follow through with such activities if there is structure, such as regularly scheduled practices or meetings.

Systematic Encouragement

As noted earlier, well-meaning clients may agree to sample a new social event, but then never reach the referral destination. To overcome potential obstacles, *Systematic Encouragement* should be utilized. It entails three recommendations: (1) Never assume that a client will make the first contact independently. Once the client agrees to try a new function, conduct a role-play of the initial phone call to the organization in the counseling session. After sufficient feedback and rehearsal, have the client make the actual phone call in the session. This provides an excellent opportunity for you to observe how the client relates to others, in addition to greatly increasing the likelihood that the client will make the call. Furthermore, it enables you to positively reinforce the client for his or her efforts. (2) Whenever possible, locate a contact person for the organization on your community resource list. Make arrangements with this person either to escort the client to the event or to meet him or her at the door. Knowing that someone is going to be there helps the client feel more comfortable about attending the activity. It also serves as a motivator to attend, since the client's intention to do so has been conveyed publicly to another person. (3) Review the experience with the client in the next session to determine the activity's reinforcement value. In other words, does the client want to attend again? Use problem-solving techniques to assist the client in overcoming any obstacles to future attendance, such as the lack of transportation or a baby sitter. In the event that the client failed to attend the activity, determine the reasons, and then engage in problem-solving.

The following example illustrates how a CRA therapist systematically encourages a client to follow through on a recreation treatment goal. The three components of the technique are noted as they occur.

THERAPIST: Susan, I think your goal of taking a country western dance class through continuing education is excellent. Let's go ahead and get you signed up.

CLIENT: I don't think I'll be able to get around to that until later in the week. I'm *really* going to be busy the next couple of days.

THERAPIST: No, I meant that we could take time right now to do it. I even have their catalog. Why don't you take a look.

Note: The therapist does not want to risk the client being "too busy" to follow through with the phone call later that week.

CLIENT: Sure. Let's see . . . here's the section on dance. There's lots of classes at night, so it won't interfere with my work schedule.

THERAPIST: Which class have you decided on?

CLIENT: This introductory class on Tuesday and Thursday evenings at seven o'clock looks good. I'll take that one.

THERAPIST: Great. Let's call right now and get you signed up before the class is full.

CLIENT: You mean call here, from your office? I'm not sure what to say.

THERAPIST: Well, Susan, we could role-play what you might say and then call. Are you comfortable with that?

CLIENT: OK. If I practice once with you I'm sure I can do it.

Note: The therapist will rehearse the phone call with the client. Feedback and verbal reinforcement will be supplied, and then the actual call will be placed.

THERAPIST: Susan, I've met the instructor for this particular dance class. Do you want me to call her and ask her to keep an eye out for you? It might be nice to have somebody watching for you.

CLIENT: I don't want to be a pain. Maybe she could just say "hello" to me when I get there, so I know I'm in the right place.

Note: Plans are made to set up a contact person. The client will feel more comfortable just knowing that someone will be watching for her. Also, she will be more likely to attend since her therapist will be informing the instructor of her intentions to do so.

THERAPIST: Fine. And we'll plan to talk about how the first two classes went when we meet next week. Now let's get to that role-play.

Note: Expectations regarding attendance are conveyed again. The therapist will check with the client in the next session to see whether she attended, and if so, whether she enjoyed it. Problem solving will be employed if needed.

Reinforcer Access

At times clients fail to develop potentially rewarding nondrinking social and recreational activities because they lack the necessary resources to participate. It may involve a shortage of money or transportation. This is particularly true of single, unemployed, socially isolated clients. Whereas Community Access procedures are designed to help clients identify and access existing community events, *Reinforcer Access* procedures are used to obtain the financial or other material prerequisites for participating in identified activities. For example, you might provide clients with a free bus pass to attend a church function, an adult education class, or a self-help group meeting. Movie passes might be distributed to the clients and their families for a rewarding "night out." Day-old newspapers could be passed along to clients so they may scan the free leisure services section.

In addition to maintaining an up-to-date, annotated community resource listing, you should be actively involved in developing reciprocal working relationships with church groups, social service agencies, and local civic and community organizations that have access to necessary financial reinforcers and transportation. Often these organizations will provide you with free or discounted tickets.

Response Priming

Initially many clients are able to reduce alcohol consumption, but for various reasons they are hesitant to become regularly involved with people and activities that support their nondrinking behavior. *Response Priming* is a technique that leads a client to take a chance on a new response activity. The "priming" refers to priming a pump so that more and more water flows. In other words, individuals will be motivated to try additional new behaviors once they have experienced success. But getting them to attempt a behavior for the first time can be a major obstacle. Response Priming addresses this issue by providing verbal or behavioral assistance at precisely the right moment. As a result, the client is in a better position to gain social support and acceptance.

In the example that follows, a client reports that she wishes she could ask a coworker to go hiking. The therapist "primes" the response by starting the sentence for the client during behavioral rehearsal and then by following it with generous reinforcement. Note that in the process the therapist is determining whether the client is hesitant because she lacks the social skills, or because she is fearful of being rejected.

CLIENT: I thought of a social activity that I'd like to ask someone to join me in: hiking. There's a guy at work, Doc, who looks like an outdoor type. Too bad I'll never have the nerve to invite him.

THERAPIST: I'm glad to hear that you're thinking of nondrinking ways to be sociable. But what do you mean when you say you'll never be able to invite him?

CLIENT: What if he gets the wrong idea and turns me down? I'd feel like an idiot!

THERAPIST: Kate, we both know that you need to find some more rewarding activities that don't involve alcohol. I don't understand the problem here. Let's role-play it.

CLIENT: No! I can't ask him! What's the use of practicing?

THERAPIST: Here, I'll get you started: Doc, I wonder if you'd be interested . . .

CLIENT: OK. OK. I'll do it. "Doc, I thought I heard you mention once that you liked hiking. I'm planning to go this Saturday morning. I always enjoy it more if I have company. Would you like to join me?"

THERAPIST: What a pro! You sounded great. You don't need any coaching from me! Now I *really* don't understand why you're reluctant to ask him.

With minimal prompting the client demonstrated in a socially skilled, assertive manner that she was capable of asking her friend to accompany her. The therapist decided that the client simply needed to be encouraged to be assertive. She did this in part by starting an "opening line" for her, and then by reinforcing her role-playing efforts. An appropriate homework assignment would follow. If the client had shown evidence of poor communication skills during the role-play, the therapist would have modeled a more appropriate response, and then rehearsed it. Feedback and reinforcement would have followed each attempt.

Response Priming has many different potential applications. But in order to target your efforts appropriately, you should first conduct a careful evaluation of the problem situation. For example, assume a client identified an interesting nondrinking function to attend (e.g., a singles dance), participated in the event (i.e., attended), but did not have any fun (i.e., get to dance). Occasionally this scenario could be the consequence of a true social skills deficit, but assume it occurred because the client simply failed to perform the entire sequence of behaviors required to obtain reinforcement (i.e., ask someone to dance). Response Priming could be used in several ways to encourage him to perform this final necessary step of asking someone to dance. You could supply him with a series of "lines" that he could use just to get started. Through role-playing he would select the most comfortable one and receive feedback on his delivery of it.

A more intense version of Response Priming would entail therapist-assisted in vivo work. Either you, a therapy assistant, or a supportive friend of the client would agree to attend a suitable social event in which the client would "try out" asking a partner to dance. During the event this "assistant" would provide continual encouragement and role-playing opportunities, until the client invited someone to dance. Afterward the assistant would review the experience with the client and use problem solving to correct any identified rough areas. Then the client would be "primed" to practice the behavior again. The assistant's prompts would be faded once the client was comfortable with performing the behavior on his own.

Social Club

Another effective method for providing clients with an opportunity to develop and practice new social skills in a non-threatening alcohol-free environment is to establish a *Social Club* similar to the one outlined by Hunt and Azrin (1973) and Mallams et al. (1982). Typically this is a weekly alcohol-free social event that is attended by clients in the recovery process. It may take place at a regular meeting hall, or the members may congregate instead at local restaurants or community events.

A Social Club offers several distinct advantages over the existing programs available in most communities: (1) Many clients are more inclined to attend Social Club rather than church or AA functions, because clients are not required to prescribe to any specific religious or recovery belief system. The only requirement is that participants in club activities are sober while attending, and that they do not bring alcohol or drugs on the premises. (2) Clients' Concerned Others are encouraged to attend all club activities as well; (3) Single, socially isolated clients can get much-needed social support and can develop nondrinking friendships at a Social Club; (4) All club functions are typically free of charge or very low in cost, and no one is refused admittance because of an inability to pay. (5) Transportation to and from club events typically is available through other club members. (6) Nutritious pot-luck meals are provided at many club activities. (7) All Social Club activities are naturally reinforcing because they are decided upon by the membership. (8) Clients and their therapists are encouraged to attend club functions together. This provides clients with the opportunity to practice new social skills, and it enables the therapist to observe clients in a real social situation. (9) Through Reinforcer Sampling the club allows clients and their Concerned Others to experience a wide variety of social interactions. Informed decisions can then be made regarding which ones are most satisfying. (10) The club serves as a "stepping-stone" back into the larger society by providing the problem drinker with a safe place to begin relating socially without the use of alcohol or drugs.

A Social Club is unique in that it does not require a great deal of initial "start-up" effort or money. Depending on members' preferences, the organization can rotate meetings between members' houses, or they can be conducted in spaces donated by local schools, church groups, hospitals, and civic organizations. Some Social Clubs have established not-for-profit corporate status and have purchased their own recreational facilities through minimal annual dues and charity drives.

♦ ♦

In summary, CRA emphasizes the importance of a healthy social and recreational life. If clients are to maintain positive changes, their new lifestyle must be more rewarding than their previous drinking lifestyle. Therefore it is imperative to learn how to motivate clients to find self-reinforcing activities, and to teach them the skills needed to access and maintain these nondrinking activities and the associated friendships.

9

CRA Marital Therapy

The marital relationship of the problem drinker is nearly always a dysfunctional one. Typically one of two scenarios is observed. Either the spouse argues with the drinker over the excessive alcohol use, or the spouse begins to withdraw, thereby decreasing the amount of communication with the drinker. Both of these situations tend to worsen over time. Given that substance abusers usually cope with tension and stress by drinking, the frequent family disputes or the spouse's withdrawn behavior begin to function as cues for the drinker to indulge in alcohol even more. Gradually a vicious cycle develops with the alcohol abuse increasing marital distress, and heightened marital conflict leading to greater alcohol abuse.

CRA emphasizes relationship counseling as an integral part of the overall approach to the treatment of alcohol abuse. Focusing exclusively on the abuser's drinking while ignoring the interpersonal problems the drinking has stemmed from or created greatly limits the benefits the problem drinker may derive from treatment. Experienced substance abuse counselors understand fully that bringing the drinker's problem under control does not necessarily result in any long-term improvement in the marital relationship. As noted, marital conflicts often were one of the reasons that the drinking escalated in the first place. If the marital situation does not improve significantly, one should anticipate that any changes in the client's drinking problem will be temporary. Consequently, helping a client combat a substance abuse problem necessarily entails improving the marital relationship. As a rule of thumb, relationship counseling should be initiated as early as possible in the treatment process.

Overview of CRA Marital Therapy

CRA's relationship counseling is action oriented and time limited. It focuses on teaching skills that can be applied to present-day problems. It views most marital conflicts as arising from unrealistic expectations, inadequate communication and problem-solving skills, and poor attempts to control the partner's behavior through aversive means. The goal of CRA's marital counseling is to teach the couple a number of general relationship skills that they then can apply to a wide range of specific interpersonal situations.

The techniques which follow are based on the early work of Nathan Azrin and Richard Stuart (Azrin, Naster, & Jones, 1973; Stuart, 1969). The modified versions that follow consist of an integrated set of behavioral and cognitive-behavioral techniques that teach couples to focus on the positive aspects of their relationship. Specialized training in goal-setting and communication skills forms the foundation of the approach.

Although called "marital" therapy, these procedures are applicable for any couple who is cohabitating or involved in a serious relationship. They can be used to solve problems between parents and adult children, heterosexual as well as homosexual couples, and in a slightly modified format, to settle relationship problems between roommates. Moreover, these procedures have been applied successfully to couples who were considering separation, or who actually already had separated as a result of one of the partner's abuse of alcohol.

Setting Positive Expectations Through CRA Marital Therapy

In many instances the distressed couples who present for therapy will have reached the point where a simple conversation has become an unpleasant event. Each individual appears to be perpetually on guard to identify and then respond to the slightest perceived negative comment or behavior of the spouse. Previously articulated complaints about an individual's behavior have long since evolved into criticisms of the individual's entire personality.

Introduce the CRA marital procedures by discussing with the

couple how their ineffective and aversive ways of communicating have created greater and greater tensions. Let them know that other couples in similarly strained relationships have improved their marriages dramatically. Inform them that you will show them how to communicate and solve their problems in a positive way in a matter of weeks. More specifically, they will learn how to make requests from their spouse in a pleasant and precise manner. They also will learn how to stop being consumed by their problems; to tackle them instead and arrive at mutually acceptable solutions. A consequence of this type of counseling is that once the partners learn to communicate more effectively, they will begin to feel that their problems are not overwhelming, and that their partner's requests are more reasonable.

A summary of the components of introducing CRA marital therapy and setting positive expectations is as follows:

1. Discuss ways the couple's current aversive communication style creates tension.
2. Assure them that other couples in similar situations have improved their relationships.
3. Explain that they will be taught communication and problem-solving skills.
4. Give specific examples of these skills, such as making requests and tackling problems together instead of dwelling on them alone.
5. Inform them that as progress is made they will feel less and less overwhelmed by their problems.
6. Discuss how the initial learning process will take weeks, not years.

MARRIAGE HAPPINESS SCALE

Description and Purpose

After CRA marital procedures have been introduced, the next step in the first marital session will differ depending on whether the client is taking disulfiram. If the individual is, the disulfiram administration procedure should be rehearsed (see Chapter 4). Each person should then be given a Marriage Happiness Scale (see Appendix 9.A). In most instances the substance-abusing client already will have completed an individual Happiness Scale (see Appendix 5.A), but the spouse will not be familiar with it. In such cases you may elect to invite the client to explain the general procedure for filling out the form. This serves two purposes. First, it boosts the client's self-image, as he or she actually is assisting you. Second, it allows you to observe how well the client understood and remembers the instructions from an earlier session. You might follow this with an illustration of the differences between the two Happiness Scales.

Both individuals should complete their scales independently, rating on a 10-point scale (1 being completely unhappy and 10 being completely happy) how satisfied or happy they presently are with *their partner* in ten important life areas. These areas include Household Responsibilities, Raising the Children, Social Activities, Money Management, Communication, Sex and Affection, Job or School, Emotional Support, and Partner's Independence. The tenth category, General Happiness, is used to provide a summary of the couples' current situation. Modifications of the first nine areas certainly are acceptable.

In the dialogue that follows, the therapist introduces the Marriage Happiness Scale to a couple. She guides them through several ratings to be certain that they fully understand the form. Discussions about potential solutions are purposely avoided at this point.

THERAPIST: Steve, you've already filled out forms pretty similar to the ones I'm going to have you and your wife complete now. But the forms you'll work on today ask about your relationship with each other instead of about individual problems and goals.

CLIENT: I've filled out a lot of forms. Which ones are we going to do?

THERAPIST: We'll start off with the couple's version of the Happiness Scale: the Marriage Happiness Scale. Let me give you each a copy.

Note: See Appendix 9.A.

THERAPIST: Let's go over the instructions. First, notice that there are ten categories listed on the left, starting with Household Responsibilities and going down through General Happiness. Each area represents an important part of a marital relationship. I'm interested in finding out today how happy each of you is with your partner in each area. So the question you each should ask yourself independently is, "How happy am I today with my partner in this area?"

CLIENT: So we don't fill this out together?

THERAPIST: No. It's important that you each complete a form on your own. I would expect that the two of you wouldn't agree on a number of the ratings at this point. So let's go ahead and take a look. Steve, you're familiar with the way the rating system works, so would you like to help explain it to Judy?

CLIENT: Sure, if I remember it right. OK. The left end of the scale is for things that you feel pretty unhappy about. Actually, the farther you go to the left, the unhappier it says you are. And the right end of the scale stands for happy feelings. So, like, a 10 rating would mean that you felt extremely happy with that area of your life.

Note: The therapist checks on the client's understanding of the scale and reinforces him accordingly.

THERAPIST: Excellent, Steve. Does that make sense, Judy?

WIFE: I think so. I'm not sure I know exactly what you mean by some of these categories, though.

THERAPIST: Well, we'll go through each one now so that there's no misunderstanding. Let's do the first one together: Household Responsibilities. Each of you should be asking yourself, "How happy am I today with my partner in the area of Household Responsibilities?" Go ahead and circle a rating. Ready? Steve, what did you circle?

CLIENT: I gave it a 9 because Judy is really good at running the house; you know, like meals, cleaning, laundry, and shopping.

THERAPIST: A 9 rating is very high, and from your description, it sounds like it's real appropriate here. Can you tell me what made you decide not to give it a 10?

CLIENT: I guess because sometimes she seems to go a little overboard with her cleaning, and then she gets really upset with me if I leave anything out at all. But I'm probably as much at fault as she is.

THERAPIST: That's fine. Your rating still seems to fit how you feel about Judy in the Household Responsibility area. Judy, what rating did you give?

WIFE: I hope I did this right. I only gave it a 7.

THERAPIST: And why don't you tell us how you arrived at that?

WIFE: Steve's not real bad about helping with the cleaning on weekends. And I don't mind doing the cooking and the laundry. Actually, I prefer doing it. But I've asked him many times to help out more during the week with little things, like washing the dishes. He never seems to get to the dishes before I do, and it upsets me.

THERAPIST: A 7 rating sounds real appropriate. Now, before we discuss strategies for making changes in some of these areas, why don't you both finish rating all of the remaining categories.

Note: At this time the therapist avoids exploring either the basis for problems raised, or solutions. The objective of this part of the session is to be certain that the couple fully understands the rating system for the Marriage Happiness Scale. The other issues will be addressed later.

THERAPIST: Judy, you mentioned you weren't sure what some of the categories meant.

WIFE: I guess it's really just the Partner's Independence one.

THERAPIST: It *is* a bit confusing. Let's first put it in the statement and proceed from there. "How happy am I today with Steve in the area of Partner's Independence?" In other words, how happy are you with *Steve's* independence, or with the amount of independence Steve shows? This could involve his independence in thinking, acting, etc.

WIFE: Oh, like do I wish he was more or less independent?

THERAPIST: Yes. You might think of things he does that you consider really independent or really dependent, and base your rating on that. Does that make sense to you now, too, Steve?

CLIENT: Yes, now it does. I would rate Judy as a 6 in that category, because she's real independent in terms of taking care of the house, but I wish she'd find some more friends. Maybe it's not my business, but I'd be happier if I saw her enjoying herself with other people sometimes, instead of waiting for me.

THERAPIST: Sounds like a good area for discussion later. Judy, how would you rate Steve's independence?

WIFE: Oh, probably a 6 too. He hangs out with his work buddies more than I'd like. Maybe he wouldn't drink so much if he spent more time at home.

The therapist covered two categories with the couple to ensure that they understood the rating system. Next she would have them complete the remaining categories and would review them briefly. Again, it is important for discussions about the issues being raised on this scale to be delayed until the entire scale is completed, and the Perfect Marriage form is introduced. (Refer to Appendixes 9.B and 9.C for examples of completed Marriage Happiness Scales.)

Potential Problems in Completing the Marriage Happiness Scale

Sometimes one member of the couple may resist becoming actively involved in working on the relationship. That person may claim to be perfectly happy with the marriage, and indicate this by marking each area on the Marriage Happiness Scale a 10. This perspective can be challenged gently in several ways. For example, you might begin by asking the couple to recall their early fantasies about marriage. Ex-

plore how the reality of the marriage is different from the fantasy. Another option is to have them think about some of their friends' happy
marriages, and to note discrepancies between their friends' marriages
and their own.

The type of resistance that involves denial of any dissatisfaction
with one's marriage occurs more frequently with the partner who is
the substance abuser. Often the underlying reason for this denial is the
fear that one's spouse might become angry and end the already shaky
relationship. It is important for you to bring these fears out in the open
so that they can be discussed.

PERFECT MARRIAGE FORM

Description and Purpose

Once the Marriage Happiness Scales have been completed and reviewed, move toward specifying the types of behavior that need to be
changed to enhance the couple's relationship. The Perfect Marriage form
is an ideal tool to facilitate this process (see Appendix 9.D). First, both
partners will be asked to complete the Perfect Marriage form independently. For each of the ten categories already introduced on the Marriage
Happiness Scale, the couple will identify behaviors in which they would
like to see their spouse engage. Agreements regarding how they will cooperate with each other to realize the desired changes will come later.

It is important for the couple to indicate all of the behaviors they
would like their partner to carry out in an ideal marriage, whether or
not they think their spouse will comply with the requests. Set the stage
for this by asking them to remember what it was like when they first
met and began dating. Have them identify the ways in which their
partner acted differently at the times when they were the happiest with
each other. Encourage them to talk about the positive aspects of their
early relationship, and the role their partner had in creating this. Tell
them that they can enjoy these good feelings again. Instruct them to
begin the process by asking for anything they want, no matter how
selfish it may seem. This "dream list" will form the foundation for later
negotiations.

Starting the Perfect Marriage Form

It is advisable to start with a category that both partners rated fairly
high on their Marriage Happiness Scales. In other words, choose an
area that already has a moderate amount of satisfaction associated with

it, and consequently requires minor changes. The goal is to have the couple leave the session feeling optimistic after having worked together actively to resolve a problem.

An illustration of using the Perfect Marriage form follows. For the first category, Household Responsibility, the form reads,

"In Household Responsibilities I would like my partner to

_____."

The client and partner are instructed to fill in the blanks by being brief and positive, and by stating in a measurable (specific) way what they would like to see their partner do. Being "positive" means phrasing requests in a way that describes those behaviors they wish their partner would perform, rather than listing those they wish he or she would *not* perform. Using "measurable" terms implies targeting the change of observable behaviors, not attitudes. You may remind the client who already has had some individual sessions that these were the rules he or she was asked to follow when setting goals and devising interventions on the Goals of Counseling form.

In the dialogue that continues you will notice the therapist shaping the couples' behavior so that it complies with the guidelines for completing the Perfect Marriage form. She also makes a point of reminding them to request whatever would really please them, regardless of whether they think their partner will comply.

THERAPIST: Let's select a category from your Marriage Happiness Scale that was rated reasonably high by both of you. That will make it easier for you to learn how to complete the form. Here are your choices of the areas you both rated pretty high: Household Responsibilities, Partner's Independence, Money Management, and Job. Where should we start?

CLIENT: We've already talked a little about the Household Responsibilities area. Maybe that's a good one. Judy?

WIFE: Sure. Sounds OK to me.

THERAPIST: Great. Judy, you indicated more dissatisfaction in this area than your husband, so let me ask you first to describe your feelings about Steve in terms of household responsibilities. Then I'll help you state your wish in a way that follows our rules.

WIFE: I think Steve forgets that I really have two jobs. One is outside the home, and the second is the stack of household chores I have to face when I get home from work. I get upset because I don't think Steve does his share. For instance, since I do the cooking, I'd like Steve to do the dishes at night.

THERAPIST: You're off to a good start. Now, there are different ways in which you can verbalize your request to Steve, but we're not going to work on that until next session. For now we'll just concentrate on writing the requests down. But we can't just write them any old way. There are certain rules we should follow, because they seem to work. The requests should be brief, positive, and specific or measurable. That's a lot! Here, I'll start you off: In the area of Household Responsibilities I would like Steve to . . . .. Now you fill in the blank with your request for him to help with the dishes. Just say it in your own words first.

Note: The therapist first invites the wife to describe the request in her own words, and then prepares to mold her response so that it adheres to the guidelines.

WIFE: I'm kind of nervous. I've never done anything like this before. What if he doesn't want to do what I ask?

THERAPIST: Don't even worry about that now. I'll help you with that next session. All we're doing today is coming up with a number of brief, positive, and specific statements. Go ahead, give it a try. You'll do fine.

Note: The therapist reminds the wife that compliance issues will be addressed later.

WIFE: How about saying I would like Steve to wash the dinner dishes at night?

THERAPIST: Good. So you'd like Steve to wash the dinner dishes at night. Let me see if I can help you be even more specific. When you say "at night," does it matter to you if he washes them at seven or eleven o'clock? If it does, then you should specify a time frame. And should we assume you mean every night?

WIFE: I would like to ask that they be done by eight o'clock. If they sit there later than that I know I'll end up washing them. I don't know about every night, though. Maybe I should just ask for help on weeknights. That's when I'm most worn out.

THERAPIST: But don't forget that this is your "dream list." You should ask for whatever would really make you happy. I'm not guaranteeing that Steve is going to agree to this. It doesn't hurt to have a little room to negotiate, though. You could always ask for his help seven nights a week, and then settle for five. The negotiating or compromising part of making and granting requests is something we'll practice next session.

Note: The therapist gradually shapes the wife's request into one that adheres to the basic rules. She reminds the wife again to ask for whatever will really make her happy, but adds that some negotiation may need to take place.

WIFE: All right. I'd like Steve to wash the dinner dishes every night before eight o'clock. How's that?

THERAPIST: Excellent. Now tell me all the rules you followed.

WIFE: I was brief, very specific, and I said it in a positive way.

THERAPIST: It sounds perfect, so I'm going to list it on your Perfect Marriage form.

Note: See Appendix 9.E, item 1.1.

Finishing the First Category on the Perfect Marriage Form

Determining who should respond first and who should respond second when completing the Perfect Marriage form during a session is a matter left to the discretion of the therapist. The decision probably will be based upon a number of factors, such as which member of the couple is less resistant, more capable, and generally more likely to serve as a good model for the partner who will proceed second. A more critical concern is that each individual has an opportunity to practice and receive feedback before leaving the session.

THERAPIST: Steve, it's your turn. What would you like to ask Judy to do in the Household Responsibilities area?

CLIENT: That's a tough one. Like I said, she's already good at this kind of thing.

THERAPIST: From what you've said, I can tell she is. But this is your dream list, Steve. What's something that Judy could do that would really make you happy?

Note: The therapist prompts the client to identify a wish, despite his reluctance to do so. Usually with the therapist's support and encouragement clients are willing and able to generate a few ideas.

CLIENT: Here's one. I would like Judy to iron my shirt for work the night before, instead of seven o'clock in the morning.

THERAPIST: Good. Can you get it to fit the rules now?

CLIENT: Should I first say why I want her to iron it at night?

THERAPIST: It's not necessary, but you're welcome to.

CLIENT: I just get nervous when she does it in the morning, because I'm afraid I'm going to end up being late for work.

THERAPIST: OK. Sounds reasonable. So how should you state the request? Fill in the blank: In the area of Household Responsibilities I would like Judy to. . . .

CLIENT: Iron my shirt for work the night before. I don't care what time it's done by, as long as it's done before bedtime. I'd like her to do it every weeknight.

THERAPIST: Go ahead and check the rules now.

CLIENT: I think I did it right. I was brief and specific, because I said every night. I guess I was positive, although I'm not really sure what it would mean to say it in a negative way.

THERAPIST: Good question. Saying something in a negative way means pointing out what someone has been doing "wrong," or saying what you *don't* want them to do. It's a way of putting your partner down a little. For example, making this request in a negative way would be saying something like, "I want Judy to stop waiting until the last minute to iron my shirt each morning." Do you see how different that sounds? It also makes it less likely that your spouse will comply with your request, because you'll be putting her on the defensive.

CLIENT: You're probably right. OK. Then I followed all the rules.

THERAPIST: I'm listing it on your Perfect Marriage form then.

Note: See Appendix 9.F, item 1.1. It should be clear from this dialogue that certain questions about following the rules only become apparent as you guide the couple through the first few examples. Depending on the degree of confusion, you would decide how many more examples should be completed during the therapy session.

THERAPIST: You both seem to be getting the knack of this. Let's do another one together in this same category of Household Responsibilities. It's your turn again, Judy.

WIFE: Hmmm. The first thing that comes to mind is the pile of dirty clothes I find on the bedroom and bathroom floors. Let's see, how should I ask him to change that? I would like Steve to throw his dirty clothes into the hamper. I'd like to ask him to always use the hamper instead of the floor, but maybe that's too much.

THERAPIST: Remember . . . dream list. Worry about negotiating later.

WIFE: Right. So I'd like Steve to always throw his dirty clothes directly into the hamper instead of onto the floor. No, that points out what I *don't* want. I guess I could just leave it at wanting him to always throw his dirty clothes directly into the hamper. There.

THERAPIST: I think you hit all the rules. You were brief, positive, and it sounded measurable. I'm putting it down on your form.

Note: See Appendix 9.E, item 1.2. With prompting, the wife proceeded to make a request for a behavior change that would bring her full satisfaction. She even corrected herself when she added a negative remark.

CLIENT: I guess it's up to me now. This is probably going to sound picky, but I'm having trouble coming up with things I'd like her to change in this area.

THERAPIST: Well, if you're already struggling to think of a request when we're only on the second one for this category, you probably wouldn't want to aim for more than two to three in the Household Responsibilities area. Although most people can come up with at least two requests in each category, I also wouldn't necessarily expect everybody to think of five all the time. But don't give up working on requests in a category until you've reminded yourself that we're talking about a "perfect" marriage.

CLIENT: True. In that case, I would like Judy to get the mending done within two weeks after something of mine has ripped, lost a button, or whatever. She has good intentions, but sometimes she forgets or gets too busy, and I'm waiting for something for two months. But I guess I shouldn't add that last negative-sounding sentence.

THERAPIST: Can you make that any more specific?

CLIENT: I don't know if this is more specific, but I actually should ask for the mending to be finished within two weeks of me telling her that something needs to be mended. I can't expect her to just know. There. Now it's brief, totally positive, and about as measurable as I can make it.

THERAPIST: Then I guess you're done. It's going on your Perfect Marriage form.

Note: See Appendix 9.F, item 1.2.

Depending on the couple's abilities, you may decide to continue rehearsing examples of requests within one category. Some CRA therapists then move on to a second category just to be certain that the procedure generalizes across topics. Have the couple work on the Perfect Marriage form for homework. Make a reasonable and specific assignment. Remember that at this stage the couple still has not been taught how to prioritize or negotiate requests. This is another set of skills that will be trained in subsequent sessions.

DAILY REMINDER TO BE NICE

In the early stages of most relationships, partners tend to exchange a large number of "pleasing" behaviors that demonstrate how much they care about each other. Sometimes it is useful to ask the couple if they remember the types of little things they used to do for each other that they do not routinely bother with now. Explain to them that they should strive for a relationship that once again maintains a higher ratio of pleasant, caring interactions than unpleasant ones.

To assist them in reestablishing a relationship that favors pleasant events, introduce the Daily Reminder to Be Nice form (see Appendix 9.G). This form lists seven general categories of "pleasing" behaviors that frequently are performed by happy couples, but rarely are found among couples in distressed relationships. The categories include expressing appreciation for something the partner does, offering compliments, giving a pleasant surprise, visibly expressing affection, devoting complete attention to a pleasant conversation, initiating pleasant conversation, and offering to help.

Ask the couple first to read through these categories to be certain that they understand how they differ from each other. Be sure the couple realizes, for example, that a compliment is not the same as an expression of appreciation. Then have them think of some behaviors in each group that would please them if their partner carried them out. Ask them to report these behaviors in brief, positive, and specific terms. Plan to shape the couple's responses and provide support. Complete several categories with them, using role-plays when appropriate. An illustration of the therapist guiding the couple through the first two categories follows.

THERAPIST: Are you both clear on expressing appreciation? It means showing gratitude or recognizing another's value. It says that you're taking nothing for granted. For example, I might say I appreciate you both attending therapy today, or I appreciate your effort to change your drinking lifestyle. So it's more than just saying something nice to somebody. Steve, could you look at Judy and express to her your appreciation for something?

CLIENT: I'm glad you came with me to this counseling session today. [Turning to the therapist] How's that?

THERAPIST: Perfect. You were brief, specific, and positive sounding. Great job. Judy, now it's your turn. Look at Steve and express your appreciation for something he did today.

WIFE: I appreciate you arranging this meeting today to fit in with my work schedule.

THERAPIST: Very good. Let's go on to the next category, complimenting your partner. We all know a compliment is an expression of praise, like telling someone they are attractive or they look especially nice in a particular outfit. But it could be something totally different from talking about how somebody looks. You could compliment your partner for a job well done, or for being clever or funny. Judy, why don't you go first this time?

WIFE: You really look handsome in that new shirt.

THERAPIST: Good job. I don't think there's any question about your message. Steve, it's your turn.

CLIENT: [Looking toward spouse] I sure did like the breakfast you made this morning. You're a good cook.

THERAPIST: Another good job by the both of you. Let's move on to the pleasant surprise category.

Note: You would continue to go down the form, making certain that the couple understands each category, and assisting them with generating examples. As usual, it is important to reinforce all of their efforts.

Once the couple understands the purpose of the Daily Reminder to Be Nice form and agrees to use it, impress upon them the importance of making a commitment to carry out specific caring behaviors *regardless* of whether their partner is doing the same. It is common among distressed couples for each one to assume that the partner should change first. Explain to them that if they each wait for the other one to act positively, nothing will happen. And as a result, each of them will become angrier and less inclined to change. So stress that each partner should agree to carry out certain positive actions during the week independent of whether or not the spouse reciprocates. Assure them that compliance problems will be addressed in the next therapy session.

Ask the couple to bring their forms to each session. This record will help you identify which individual shows a greater willingness to take constructive action. The spouse who appears less motivated may require the greater therapeutic effort and support. Upon returning home the couple should post the Daily Reminder to Be Nice form in a prominent location, such as on the refrigerator door or the bathroom mirror.

Summary of First Session Accomplishments

Frequently CRA therapists end the first marital session at this point. The following have been accomplished:

1. Relationship problems have been pointed out, and the rationale for couples' counseling has been introduced.
2. CRA's approach to couples' counseling has been presented.
3. Positive expectations have been set.

4. The disulfiram administration procedure has been explained and rehearsed (if applicable).
5. The Marriage Happiness Scale has been introduced and completed.
6. The Perfect Marriage form has been presented, and the instructions and rules have been reviewed and practiced.
7. The Daily Reminder to Be Nice form has been explained and tested.
8. Specific homework assignments to continue working with the forms have been made.

Often the first marital session proves to be a relatively pleasant experience for the couple. This may be due to several factors: (1) In some cases the drinker starts taking disulfiram, at which point the person gains self-confidence. In turn, this enables the spouse to see that the drinker is committed to changing, and consequently both trust and hope are reintroduced. (2) The overall atmosphere of the marital session is very positive. Complaints and blaming are kept to a minimum, and requests for behavior change are always stated in positive terms. (3) Problems that appear overwhelming at the onset are broken down into smaller, manageable parts, and specific skills for dealing with these more manageable problems are identified. As a result, the couple tends to leave the session with a more optimistic attitude.

It is important to schedule the second marital session to take place shortly after the first. If possible, do not allow more than 3 to 4 days to pass. Keeping in close contact with the couple is essential at the beginning of the therapeutic relationship. Initially any changes the partners make are tenuous at best. More frequent sessions at this stage in treatment help the couple to overcome barriers and accelerate positive changes in their relationship.

Subsequent Sessions

There are several tasks that should be accomplished in subsequent CRA marital therapy sessions:

1. Have the couple perform the disulfiram administration procedure (if applicable). This affords an opportunity to provide corrective feedback if necessary, and as always, reinforcement for their efforts.
2. Ask the couple to complete a new Marriage Happiness Scale. This will allow you to monitor progress on an ongoing basis.

Any noteworthy rating changes in either direction from the previous week's should be queried. In this manner newly introduced or exacerbated problems may be added to the session's agenda, and improvements may be noted and reinforced.

3. Review the Daily Reminder to Be Nice forms. Ask how each partner felt about both performing the behaviors they reported, and being the recipient of their partner's caring acts. Discuss whether they want assistance in modifying any of the behaviors that are designed to please the partner, or in generating ideas for additional behaviors.

4. Resume work on the Perfect Marriage forms. Assist the couple in identifying additional behavior changes they would like to see in their spouse.

5. Remind the couple of new skills that were taught the previous week (e.g., problem solving), and ask them to demonstrate the skills in a role-play. Reinforce any attempt, and shape the behavior as needed.

At this point in the session a particular tone will be set, usually depending on how compliant each spouse was with the homework during the week. If both individuals made genuine efforts to work on the relationship, an optimistic mood will prevail. You would then proceed to the new agenda for the session, which early in therapy might entail refining and verbally practicing requests from the Perfect Marriage form. On the other hand, if one or both partners neither attempted to complete the assignment nor showed any signs of interacting positively, you should turn your attention to discovering the basis for the resistance to change.

Handling Ambivalence About Changing

In dealing with the problem of incomplete homework assignments, it is important to address the issue without dwelling upon it. Explore the reasons for the noncompliance, but always in a manner that focuses primarily on eliminating obstacles that could interfere with completing assignments the next week. In the course of this discussion it may become apparent that the couple has been experiencing ambivalence about making changes in their relationship. These feelings should be acknowledged, and the fact that it often is "easier" to maintain the status quo despite the unhappiness it has created should be explored.

Sometimes it is useful to ask the couple whether they are willing to invest a few weeks of hard work in their relationship for the potential payoff of a much happier marriage. The most they have to lose is some wasted effort. Then, without blaming either partner, point out that significant changes will be realized only through the combined effort of both individuals. In part, this involves both spouses completing their segment of the agreed-upon homework assignments. While at times the tasks may seem trivial, explain that the small daily changes lay the foundation for positive emotions and reestablished trust in the relationship.

The Basics of Positive Communication Skills

Before describing the actual components of a good conversation, present a rationale for working on communication skills. Explain how the client's drinking problem has contributed to the deterioration of the couple's ability to communicate with each other. Encourage them to supply specific examples of this process as it has unfolded over time. Explore with them whether their frustrations and distress have grown to the point where they have stopped making the effort to be friendly to each other.

Sometimes one or both individuals report being reluctant to attempt any kind of positive communication, because they actively feel angry with their spouse. They insist that it would be hypocritical to speak pleasantly when they feel resentful. If this occurs, make it clear that changes in behavior often precede changes in attitudes and feelings toward one's partner. Ultimately, most couples will agree that they have little to lose by attempting to communicate pleasantly with each other for a week.

As you prepare to describe the components of good communication skills, inform the couple that, in the process of completing the Perfect Marriage form, they already have worked on several basic communication skills in at least one area: making requests. Point out that they will be satisfying the first three guidelines for a good conversation if they just follow the rules for completing that form. The basic components are as follows:

1. Briefly present one issue.
2. Speak in a positive manner, and avoid all blaming statements.
3. Define the issue clearly and specifically.
4. State your feelings about the issue.
5. Try to view the issue from your partner's perspective, and offer an understanding statement to that effect.
6. Accept partial responsibility for any problem raised, instead of viewing your partner as totally at fault.
7. Offer to help in the situation.

Be sure to list the seven positive communication steps on a blackboard, or provide a handout. Alert the couple to the fact that the steps may vary slightly, depending on the purpose of the interaction.

Practicing Requests with the Perfect Marriage Form

The couple introduced earlier in this chapter has returned for their second session. Recall that they completed part of the Perfect Marriage form with the therapist during the first session. In addition they finished several sections as part of a homework assignment. Assume that the therapist has reviewed their work and offered feedback and reinforcement. She also has outlined the basic components of good communication skills, and is prepared to help the couple rehearse one specific, practical application: making and negotiating verbal requests.

THERAPIST: Next we're going to use some of the entries you made on your Perfect Marriage forms to practice verbalizing those requests. You've done lots of the work already by following the three rules when writing your requests. Now I'll show you how to apply the basic communication skills I just outlined to some real-life situations. I thought we could begin with the main category you've been working on: Household Responsibilities. So Steve, why don't you start us off by making a positive request from your wife in the Household Responsibility area? Look at your Perfect Marriage form and decide which request you'd like to make first. Then go ahead and simply read it out loud. That's a good place to start, because you've already stated it in a way that's specific, positive, and brief.

CLIENT: Here goes. I'm going to ask for the first one I listed. Judy, I would like you to iron my shirt for work every weeknight before bedtime.

THERAPIST: Don't answer him yet. We need to work on the way Steve is presenting his request to you. So let's turn to our list of things to include in a good communication. By adding some of these other points, Steve, you'll increase the chance of Judy agreeing to your request.

Note: Refer to the seven basic components of good communication skills (p. 163).

CLIENT: But I'm not going to have this list with me when I talk to her outside of these sessions. How am I supposed to remember all of the things I need to include?

THERAPIST: I'm glad you brought that up. You're right. Normally you won't be carrying these rules and forms around with you. But if you practice with them during our sessions and the next couple of weeks at home, you'll remember enough of the rules to make a big improvement in how you talk to each other.

So far the therapist selected a category that should be a relatively easy one to practice, and instructed the client to begin verbalizing a request by reading it directly from the Perfect Marriage form. Then she addressed the issue of carefully following the rules and using the forms during the early stages of therapy, so that eventually new skills would be automatic and forms would be unnecessary.

Enhancing the Basic Request with New Communication Skills

The therapist is ready to build upon the basic request that already appears on the Perfect Marriage form. Step-by-step the new communication skills (items 4–7, p. 163) will be introduced and rehearsed. Then the final version of the request will be presented.

THERAPIST: Go ahead and read your request again, Steve. And then we'll take it from there.

CLIENT: Sure. Judy, I would like you to iron my shirt for work every weeknight before bedtime.

THERAPIST: Now watch. You'll be surprised to see how many of the "good communication skills" points you've already covered. You briefly presented only one issue, you said it in a positive way without blaming, and you defined it clearly and specifically. So the first three are done. Now here's the new part. Can you state your feelings about why it's important to you that Judy try to iron your shirt at night? As a matter of fact, I think you even mentioned it last week when you first brought up this request.

CLIENT: I did. Sure. I get real nervous if she irons in the morning because I'm afraid I'm going to be late for work. There's a lot of commotion in our house before work and school, and sometimes she has to really rush to finish my shirt.

THERAPIST: That's perfect, Steve. You said that it made you feel nervous and you explained why. Now, can you do #5: Try to view the issue from your partner's perspective, and offer an understanding statement?

CLIENT: Well, I definitely understand that it's hard for Judy to have time to get the shirt ironed at all, because she's got so much else to do.

THERAPIST: Good. That's your "understanding statement" right there.

Here's an interesting one now. Can you accept partial responsibility for the problem that you've brought up?

CLIENT: Let me think. Yes, because if I did the dishes at night, like I know she's going to ask me to do, she'd have time to do the ironing at night.

THERAPIST: Beautifully said. One more point to go. Can you offer to help in some way?

CLIENT: I suppose the obvious thing would be to offer to help with the dishes more.

Note: Next the therapist will ask the client to put all the pieces of the conversation together. Not only will this provide additional practice in composing a good conversation, but it also will allow the partner to hear the full request in an uninterrupted manner. Typically the polished version of the request elicits a much more favorable response.

THERAPIST: Go ahead now and put it altogether so we can see how it sounds. I'll remind you of the new rules, or you can refer to the paper where I wrote them down for you.

CLIENT: I'll read the section off the form first. Judy, I would like you to iron my shirt for work every weeknight before bedtime. OK. Now the new parts: Judy, it makes me nervous when you iron my shirt in the morning, because you're so busy trying to do so many things that I'm afraid you might run out of time. Then I'd be late for work.

THERAPIST: You're doing terrific, Steve. Two more sentences to add. Can you accept partial responsibility, and offer to help?

CLIENT: Right. Judy, I guess I don't help matters much, because you'd probably have more time to do things like ironing at night if I freed you up by doing more around the house. So how about I do my share and help with the dishes more?

THERAPIST: I think that sounds good, Steve, but what's more important is how Judy thinks it sounds.

The Role of the Listener

The most "perfect" type of communication will never be utilized if it continually fails to elicit the desired response from the partner. This does not necessarily mean that the partner has to agree to every request, but he or she should at least listen attentively and ask for clarification when needed. The final "rule" for the listener is to never refuse a request outright, but instead to offer an alternative.

THERAPIST: So what do you think, Judy?

WIFE: It's funny, because when he first said that he wanted to ask me to iron his shirts at night, I got sort of upset; like he was putting another demand on me. But when I hear him say it the way he is now, it doesn't really upset me. I'm not sure I'm ready to go along with it yet, but I know I could talk to him about it.

THERAPIST: That's exactly where you should be right now; ready to talk or maybe even negotiate. But before we do that, let me just check with you on a few things. Did you listen attentively, and do you need to ask Steve to clarify what he's asking you to do?

WIFE: I listened to everything he said. The only thing that's not clear is how much he's willing to do in return, and how often.

THERAPIST: It sounds like you're entertaining the idea of trying to honor Steve's request, but you need to negotiate the terms a little so that it can happen. Right?

WIFE: Yes. And he's already said that he doesn't help enough.

THERAPIST: Good. You're bringing up one of those unwritten "rules," which says it's best to never refuse a request outright, but to offer an alternative. Maybe you'd like to negotiate right now. It would really be like making a bargain. You'll iron his shirt at night if _____. You fill it in.

WIFE: I'd like to ask him to help me out by doing the dishes after dinner. Actually, that's the exact request I listed first on my Perfect Marriage form. I was going to ask him to do it anyway! Now if he agrees to do it, he gets something in return.

It is fairly common for one partner's response to a request to be somewhat contingent upon how well a request of his or her own is received. Although communications of this type are slightly more complicated, the same guidelines apply.

The Art of Negotiation

It is imperative that the partner be given the opportunity to consider a request fully, and to respond in a manner that is completely acceptable to him or her. Otherwise the individual may verbally agree to a request in the session, but harbor resentment. The likelihood of the request actually being honored in such a case is remote. So the therapist invites the wife in the scenario to negotiate the husband's request by offering one of her own.

THERAPIST: Steve, it sounds like you're not going to get a final answer from Judy until she finds out how willing you are to do something for her. Judy, go ahead and state your request to Steve the way it's written on your form. Then we'll work on adding the points that make it sound even better.

WIFE: Steve, I would like you to wash the dinner dishes every night before eight o'clock. And now I add the next part, starting with number 4?

THERAPIST: Go right ahead. Holler if you need help.

WIFE: Steve, I'm really tired when I get home from work, and I know you're exhausted, too, because you've always been a hard worker, but it would really show me that you care. Wait, I'm stuck! Accepting partial responsibility. I'm not sure about that one. I mean, I suppose I could accept partial responsibility for the dishes being dirty, but I don't think that's what you mean by that point.

THERAPIST: Accepting partial responsibility is really just another way of *not* blaming your spouse, or of *not* implying that the whole problem is his fault. It's a way of saying that you play a part in the problem, just like he does.

WIFE: Maybe I could say that I wish I had more energy after dinner like I used to. It never bothered me that much before. I always did the dishes and never said anything. I can see why he got used to it. Does that sound like I'm accepting some of the responsibility?

THERAPIST: Yes. And you're even offering a second understanding statement. I was going to suggest something along the line of accepting partial responsibility for not getting the table cleared and the dishes stacked fast enough. I don't know whether that applies in your case, but if it did it would be a good example of accepting partial responsibility.

WIFE: No, I don't think that's part of the problem, because I clear the table pretty fast usually.

Note: There are many different ways in which one can accept partial responsibility. It can be approached from the angle of accepting partial responsibility for the problem existing in the first place, or for a solution not being attempted. Regardless, the main objective is for couples to get into the habit of never viewing their partner as totally at fault for a problem. Instead, each individual should be willing to accept the fact that they played a role themselves.

THERAPIST: Last thing: Can you offer to help?

CLIENT: Hmmm. That's a tough one, because I already feel like I'm doing most of the work at home. Would it count if I just offered not to bug him about the dishes up until eight o'clock? I'd really prefer to have them done sooner, but if we agreed to this deadline I could try hard not to say anything about the dishes before then.

THERAPIST: Sounds like a good offer. Nice job. Let's see what Steve's reaction is. But first, were you listening carefully, Steve?

CLIENT: I didn't miss a word!

THERAPIST: Do you need to have Judy explain what she meant by her request?

CLIENT: Only the part you just brought up! Who would be clearing the table? I assumed she would, like always, but now I'm not so sure.

WIFE: No, I wouldn't mind still clearing the table and stacking the dishes. I'd be happy if you just washed them.

THERAPIST: Then it's time to make a decision. Should you agree to her request, or offer an alternative? It's a little complicated, because you're both making requests at the same time. Can you figure out a way you both get what you want?

Note: The therapist has just reviewed the "listener's" part. Now she sees if the couple can negotiate the final solution on their own, or whether they will need assistance with the process.

WIFE: How about this? I'll agree to iron Steve's shirts at night if he washes the dishes on those same nights. In other words, I'll even change my request to just five nights a week so we're both doing something nice for each other on the same nights. What do you say, Steve?

CLIENT: Sounds good to me. I know I need to help you out more around the house, and like you said before, this way I even get something I really want in return.

THERAPIST: So you've agreed to each other's requests?

CLIENT: Looks like it.

THERAPIST: That's something to be proud of. And I hope after we do a few more of these in here, you'll be eager to try this kind of communication process on your own. Can we all agree that you'll try this new arrangement for a week? We can talk at our next session about any problems you ran into.

The therapist sets an expectation that each partner will carry out their new task for the week. She also informs them that certain difficulties may arise, but that they will be addressed in the next session. Since the new tasks are sizeable and will be attempted five days out of the seven, the therapist will not ask the couple to make another household request of each other. She may, however, have them practice verbalizing a small request from a different category. Also, she probably will ask them to write down their tasks on a piece of paper that can be posted at home as a reminder.

In subsequent sessions when checking on follow-through, you may discover that some couples respond better to requests that include built-in sanctions for noncompliance. For instance, assume a husband has agreed to take out the trash if it is placed by the door in plastic bags. He has also agreed that if he forgets to do so, he then will make supper for one night in addition to taking out the trash. Try variations on this theme, and discover whatever seems to work best and is comfortable for each individual couple.

Ending the Session

Before ending any session be sure to positively reinforce all the work the couple has done to this point, and assure them that things will continue to improve. Remind them to work on their assignments during the week and to bring their forms to the next session. Finally, encourage them to call if they are having any problems between appointments. Beyond the first few couples' sessions, the remaining ones usually are scheduled weekly.

♦ ♦

In summary, this chapter presented a rationale for working on the marital relationship of a problem drinker and offered a solid format for doing so. Provisions for monitoring progress were included by the introduction of the Marriage Happiness Scale. Basic communication skills were trained through both written (Perfect Marriage form) and verbal (making requests) tasks. The primary emphasis throughout was on treating one's partner in a positive, respectful manner. This was evidenced by many of the rules for good communication, as well as the reliance upon such procedures as completing the Daily Reminder to Be Nice form.

APPENDIX 9.A   *MARRIAGE HAPPINESS SCALE*

This scale is intended to estimate your current happiness with your marriage in each of the ten areas listed below. Ask yourself the following question as you rate each area:

"How happy am I today with my partner in this area?"

Then circle the number that applies. Numbers toward the left indicate various degrees of unhappiness, while numbers toward the right reflect various levels of happiness.

In other words, by using the proper number you will be indicating just how happy you are with that particular marriage area.

Remember: You are indicating your current happiness, that is, how you feel today. Also, try not let your feelings in one area influence the ratings in another area.

	Completely unhappy									Completely happy
Household Responsibilities	1	2	3	4	5	6	7	8	9	10
Raising the Children	1	2	3	4	5	6	7	8	9	10
Social Activities	1	2	3	4	5	6	7	8	9	10
Money Management	1	2	3	4	5	6	7	8	9	10
Communication	1	2	3	4	5	6	7	8	9	10
Sex & Affection	1	2	3	4	5	6	7	8	9	10
Job or School	1	2	3	4	5	6	7	8	9	10
Emotional Support	1	2	3	4	5	6	7	8	9	10
Partner's Independence	1	2	3	4	5	6	7	8	9	10
General Happiness	1	2	3	4	5	6	7	8	9	10

Name:_____

Date:_____

APPENDIX 9.B *MARRIAGE HAPPINESS SCALE*

This scale is intended to estimate your current happiness with your marriage in each of the ten areas listed below. Ask yourself the following question as you rate each area:

"How happy am I today with my partner in this area?"

Then circle the number that applies. Numbers toward the left indicate various degrees of unhappiness, while numbers toward the right reflect various levels of happiness.

In other words, by using the proper number you will be indicating just how happy you are with that particular marriage area.

Remember: You are indicating your current happiness, that is, how you feel today. Also, try not let your feelings in one area influence the ratings in another area.

	Completely unhappy									Completely happy
Household Responsibilities	1	2	3	4	5	6	(7)	8	9	10
Raising the Children	1	2	3	4	(5)	6	7	8	9	10
Social Activities	1	2	(3)	4	5	6	7	8	9	10
Money Management	1	2	3	4	5	(6)	7	8	9	10
Communication	1	2	3	(4)	5	6	7	8	9	10
Sex & Affection	1	2	(3)	4	5	6	7	8	9	10
Job or School	1	2	3	4	5	(6)	7	8	9	10
Emotional Support	1	2	(3)	4	5	6	7	8	9	10
Partner's Independence	1	2	3	4	5	(6)	7	8	9	10
General Happiness	1	2	3	(4)	5	6	7	8	9	10

Name: *Judy*

Date: *6/1*

APPENDIX 9.C *MARRIAGE HAPPINESS SCALE*

This scale is intended to estimate your current happiness with your marriage in each of the ten areas listed below. Ask yourself the following question as you rate each area:

"How happy am I today with my partner in this area?"

Then circle the number that applies. Numbers toward the left indicate various degrees of unhappiness, while numbers toward the right reflect various levels of happiness.

In other words, by using the proper number you will be indicating just how happy you are with that particular marriage area.

Remember: You are indicating your current happiness, that is, how you feel today. Also, try not let your feelings in one area influence the ratings in another area.

	Completely unhappy									Completely happy
Household Responsibilities	1	2	3	4	5	6	7	8	(9)	10
Raising the Children	1	2	3	4	5	6	7	(8)	9	10
Social Activities	1	2	3	4	5	(6)	7	8	9	10
Money Management	1	2	3	4	5	6	(7)	8	9	10
Communication	1	2	3	4	5	6	(7)	8	9	10
Sex & Affection	1	2	3	4	5	(6)	7	8	9	10
Job or School	1	2	3	4	5	6	7	(8)	9	10
Emotional Support	1	2	3	4	(5)	6	7	8	9	10
Partner's Independence	1	2	3	4	5	(6)	7	8	9	10
General Happiness	1	2	3	4	5	6	(7)	8	9	10

Name: *Steve*

Date: *6/1*

APPENDIX 9.D   *PERFECT MARRIAGE*

Under each area listed below, write down what activities would occur in what would be for *you* an ideal marriage. Be brief, be positive, and state in a specific and measurable way what you would like to occur.

1. In Household Responsibilities I would like my partner to:

   1._____

   2._____

   3._____

   4._____

   5._____

2. In Raising the Children I would like my partner to:

   1._____

   2._____

   3._____

   4._____

   5._____

3. In Social Activities I would like my partner to:

   1._____

   2._____

   3._____

   4._____

   5._____

4. In Money Management I would like my partner to:

1._____

2._____

3._____

4._____

5._____

5. In Communication I would like my partner to:

1._____

2._____

3._____

4._____

5._____

6. In Sex and Affection I would like my partner to:

1._____

2._____

3._____

4._____

5._____

7. In Job or School I would like my partner to:

1._____

2._____

3._____

4._____

5._____

8. In Emotional Support I would like my partner to:

1._____

2._____

3._____

4._____

5._____

9. In Partner's Independence I would like my partner to:

1._____

2._____

3._____

4._____

5._____

10. In General Happiness I would like my partner to:

1._____

2._____

3._____

4._____

5._____

APPENDIX 9.E *PERFECT MARRIAGE*

Under each area listed below, write down what activities would occur in what would be for *you* an ideal marriage. Be brief, be positive, and state in a specific and measurable way what you would like to occur.

1. In Household Responsibilities I would like my partner to:

   1. *Wash the dinner dishes every night before 8:00*

   2. *Always throw his dirty clothes directly into the hamper*

   3. _____

   4. _____

   5. _____

2. In Raising the Children I would like my partner to:

   1. _____

   2. _____

   3. _____

   4. _____

   5. _____

3. In Social Activities I would like my partner to:

   1. _____

   2. _____

   3. _____

   4. _____

   5. _____

APPENDIX 9.F   *PERFECT MARRIAGE*

Under each area listed below, write down what activities would occur in what would be for *you* an ideal marriage. Be brief, be positive, and state in a specific and measurable way what you would like to occur.

1. In Household Responsibilities I would like my partner to:

   1. *Iron my shirt for work every weeknight before bedtime*

   2. *Get the mending done within 2 weeks of me telling her*

   3. _____

   4. _____

   5. _____

2. In Raising the Children I would like my partner to:

   1. _____

   2. _____

   3. _____

   4. _____

   5. _____

3. In Social Activities I would like my partner to:

   1. _____

   2. _____

   3. _____

   4. _____

   5. _____

APPENDIX 9.G   *DAILY REMINDER TO BE NICE*

Name: _____

Week Starting: _____

Day of Week							
Did you express appreciation to your partner today?							
Did you compliment your partner today?							
Did you give your partner any pleasant surprises today?							
Did you visibly express affection to your partner today?							
Did you spend some time devoting your complete attention to pleasant conversation with your partner?							
Did you initiate any of the pleasant conversations?							
Did you make any offer to help before being asked?							

179

10

CRA Relapse Prevention

Today all solid substance abuse programs include a relapse component. CRA's relapse prevention begins with the first session and is a constant process. The functional analysis already was introduced as a tool that outlines the antecedents and consequences of common drinking episodes. It also can be adapted to trace a single relapse episode with the objective of preventing a recurrence. This chapter will use the functional analysis and several other methods to illustrate how an individual begins to drink again as the result of a sequence of identifiable decisions. The goal will be to learn how to *prevent* unwanted drinking altogether, and how to *intervene* in the event that it occurs.

Functional Analysis: Relapse Version

CRA utilizes a separate functional analysis form for a single relapse episode. In this way you can break down the relapse into minute detail and show more precisely what caused it. The dialogue that follows illustrates how to use the CRA Functional Analysis for Drinking Behavior (Relapse Version) form (Appendix 10.A) to prevent future relapses. The therapist begins the session by reinforcing the client for returning to treatment at such a difficult time. She immediately adopts a solution orientation (see Chapter 7) and moves the client in a problem-solving direction. The connection between the client's drinking triggers and his relapse is highlighted. Alternatives to drinking during that stressful, high-risk period are generated next. And finally, the therapist checks to see that the short-term positive consequences associated with the drinking episode are also obtainable through the identified alternative behavior. This increases the probability that the client will actually consider the alternative behavior in a future high-risk circumstance.

THERAPIST: Rafael, it's good to see you again. I'm sorry to hear you've been having trouble, but I'm glad you came in. What's going on?

CLIENT: I got laid off my job and just started to drink again. I had that job for ten years. It really kills me.

THERAPIST: That's horrible. Is there any chance to get your job back?

CLIENT: No, they shut the plant down.

THERAPIST: We have a Job Finding Program here. I think it would be a good idea for you to see our job counselor and get started looking for a new job as soon as possible.

Note: The therapist reinforces the client for returning to therapy after a relapse. She continues to move the session in a positive direction by suggesting that the client contact the Job Finding Program.

CLIENT: Yes, I'll do that. I want to work. I need the money. I have a car payment and a mortgage.

THERAPIST: I'll introduce you to our job counselor right after our session. But right now I'd like to take a close look at your relapse. Do you remember how when we first started we filled out a chart that showed triggers and consequences to drinking?

CLIENT: Yes. We did it the first time we met. What about it?

THERAPIST: Well, I want to do another chart very similar to that one. This chart is intended to analyze the relapse so we can prevent another one from occurring.

CLIENT: I know why I drank; I got laid off. I'm mad! It's unfair!

THERAPIST: It *is* unfair, and I know you have strong feelings about it. So let's take those feelings; some of the ones that probably led up to drinking, and put them on the chart. Let's start from the top at the left hand corner and go from there.

Note: Refer to the CRA Functional Analysis for Drinking Behavior (Relapse Version) form (Appendix 10.A).

CLIENT: I was with my brother-in-law, Max. He got laid off, too. Should I just go ahead and answer the next question?

THERAPIST: Keep going. You're doing great.

CLIENT: We drank mostly at his house. He lives alone so there was no one to hassle us. We've been drinking beer since last Friday, the day we were laid off. So I've been drinking almost steady for 5 days.

Note: The client has supplied information on all the external triggers. The therapist completed the first column. Refer to the completed chart (Appendix 10.B).

THERAPIST: I'm glad you decided to stop. It must have been hard. Let's see how we can prevent further problems. Let's go on to the second column. What were you thinking about just before you started to drink?

CLIENT: I was thinking how unfair it was to be laid off. I was just plain mad.

THERAPIST: So you were thinking about how unfair it was to be laid off.

CLIENT: That's right. They lied to us and then just threw us out. I felt *sick*. I mean physically sick.

THERAPIST: What do you mean you felt physically sick?

CLIENT: My stomach got upset. And I felt tense and wanted to ease down; to take away the pressure. I felt more hurt and angry than anything. So I got wasted. I deserved a good drunk. I got laid off.

THERAPIST: So the way you handled these problems was to drink.

CLIENT: That's right. I'd been sober for 6 months. I deserved it. I got laid off.

Note: Column #2, "Internal Triggers", is now complete. At this point it is easy to see how negative emotional states, negative self-talk, and poor coping skills all played into the relapse.

THERAPIST: I'm sure you're feeling very upset and cheated because of the layoff. But there are other ways you could have handled this problem. Drinking is not the best solution. In a minute we'll see how something like problem solving could have helped. But let's finish examining the relapse episode first. If you look at the chart, you can see that in column #3 you have already answered most of the questions. You stated earlier that you were drinking beer with your brother-in-law for the last 5 days. How much would you guess you drank?

CLIENT: We went through about a case a day, so I probably had half of that; about 2½ to 3 cases altogether.

THERAPIST: What were some of the immediate positive things that came out of the drinking?

CLIENT: Well, we went on and on about us both being laid off. I like hanging out with Max. And I like his place because we can drink in peace.

THERAPIST: Good, go on!

CLIENT: I felt good when we started drinking, mostly because we were putting down the company. It made me feel good; even satisfied. Like we were getting revenge. But then it was hard to stop.

THERAPIST: What about any pleasant physical feelings?

CLIENT: It made me feel kind of relaxed, I guess.

THERAPIST: How could you tell you were relaxed?

CLIENT: My stomach settled down. It didn't feel all knotted up anymore.

Note: The therapist has finished gathering information for column #3: "Behavior," and column #4, "Short-Term Positive Consequences." Next, she may either continue with the chart and outline the long-term negative consequences of drinking or decide to inquire about alternative behaviors that also could have given the client those positive short-term consequences. You simply decide based on whatever you think would be most beneficial to the particular client. This therapist opted to raise the issue of alternative, nondrinking behaviors.

THERAPIST: Rafael, it's obvious that the drinking gave you a number of important things that you felt you really needed at the time. But I bet there were other things, nondrinking things, that you could have done that would have given you those same pleasant thoughts and feelings. Can you think of any?

CLIENT: I've thought about it. I know we worked on this weeks ago. I suppose I could have started by going home and telling my wife. Or maybe I should have stopped at an AA meeting first. I wonder if Max would have gone to an AA meeting with me?

THERAPIST: Those all sound like decent ideas. Which one do you think would have been the best choice for you at the time? Remember, you wanted to be with someone you liked in a comfortable place. You wanted to be able to talk a lot about how angry you were about the layoff. You mentioned getting some satisfaction out of talking, and then feeling relaxed afterwards.

Note: The therapist is going down the list of responses provided by the client in the column marked "Short-Term Positive Consequences" of drinking. If the alternative behavior does not provide these same positive effects, then the chances of the client relying on that behavior in the future are slim.

CLIENT: I think I should have brought Max to a meeting with me. Then I could have taken him home with me to dinner. My wife wouldn't of minded.

THERAPIST: And do you think you would have gotten what you needed at that time?

CLIENT: Probably. It makes a lot of sense now.

THERAPIST: What would have been the advantages to handling your feelings by going to a meeting with Max and then home to dinner, instead of drinking for five days?

CLIENT: I may not have gotten drunk at all. I know I'm impulsive, and if I could have cooled it for a day or two I might have made it. I was just so angry I flew off the handle.

THERAPIST: It's OK, Rafael. You are doing the right thing now by initiating therapy again to stop the drinking. We'll continue with the problem solving in just a few minutes. Right now I'd like to finish the relapse chart. Let's look at the last column: "Long-Term Negative Consequences."

CLIENT: Do you want me to go down the list or just talk about the negative stuff?

THERAPIST: Sure. Just talk about it.

CLIENT: Well, my wife is real angry, and so are my parents. I feel sick and like a failure. The rest is easy to figure out. I need a job.

THERAPIST: Did the 5 days of drinking hurt your job situation or your finances in any way?

CLIENT: I spent money on beer that I really didn't have to spare. My job? Well, I suppose I could have been out looking for a new one, or at least getting some ideas.

THERAPIST: You've done a good job here today, Rafael. Let's take an in-depth look at your relapse using the chart. Then we'll use problem solving to find better ways for handling your crises.

Refer to Appendix 10.B to see how the therapist completed the last column with this information. The therapist next would use the relapse chart to summarize and instruct. She would review the triggers in detail to show the client where he made costly decisions. Then clinical procedures, including cognitive restructuring and problem solving, would be introduced again to train appropriate ways to cope. She would use the relapse as a model to help the client learn better ways to make decisions.

The Behavioral Chain Leading to Relapse

One of the new skills taught within CRA is learning to recognize when temptation is building or a slip is close. Slips typically do not occur in response to just one trigger, but after a sequence of triggers. This set of events is called a Behavioral Chain. The characters and the situation in the dialogue just presented will be used now to illustrate how to review with a client the series of decisions and events that led directly to his relapse. You may choose to use a blackboard to show Rafael in black and white how the relapse began to unfold long before he sipped his first drink.

Step 1. Rafael feels angry and cheated. He wants to know how Max is handling the layoff.

Step 2. He leaves work and drives toward Max's house. He still believes he just wants to hear what Max thinks about the whole thing.

Step 3. He feels anxious the closer he gets to Max's house.

Step 4. He enters Max's house with an uncomfortable feeling. The atmosphere elicits old feelings associated with drinking.

Step 5. Rafael and Max sit down in the kitchen and start to put down the company. Their voices get louder and louder.

Step 6. Max starts to pace around the room saying he's thirsty.

Step 7. Max searches through the refrigerator and pulls out two bottles of beer.

Step 8. Max places a beer in front of Rafael on the table.

Step 9. Max pushes the beer toward Rafael while telling him he needs to cool off.

Step 10. Rafael accepts the offer and begins to drink.

This series of events points out how Rafael's decision to see how Max was handling the layoff started the relapse process. You would show Rafael how he made a small decision at each step along the way that led him further and further in the direction of drinking. For example, when Max began pacing and said he was thirsty (Step 6), Rafael *decided* to remain seated at the table. A safer decision would have been either to get up and leave at that point, or to say that he could not hang around with Max anymore that night if he was going to drink. You also would make it clear that it typically is much easier to interrupt a behavioral chain early, as opposed to later, in the process. For instance, it would have been easier for Rafael to resist the temptation to drink that evening if he had decided to see how one of his nondrinking friends was handling the layoff (Step 1), instead of going to Max's house. The decision *not* to drink would have been much more difficult if Rafael had tried to make it once he already was in a familiar old drinking setting: Max's kitchen (Step 5).

A behavioral chain can be introduced in a number of different places during a session that is dealing with a relapse. You may choose to illustrate the sequence of events that led to a relapse at the point that the triggers are being outlined, or after the entire functional analysis for the relapse episode has been completed.

Early Warning System

Both the CRA Functional Analysis (Relapse Version) and the behavioral chain exercise just illustrated are tools best suited for a therapist and client working together *after* a relapse already has taken place. For relapse *prevention* work, some therapists rely on the triggers section of the initial functional analysis to help clients foresee upcoming high risk situations. Others prefer a simpler tool: the *Early Warning System*.

The Early Warning System is a specific relapse prevention self-monitoring procedure designed to track the behaviors of clients that appear to be the antecedents, or triggers, to drinking. The system is most successful when a Concerned Other is trained in the procedure along with the client. In addition to providing valuable input regarding drinking triggers, the Concerned Other can often recognize the earliest signs of an impending relapse before the client.

As part of the training for the Early Warning System, the client and the Concerned Other agree to assist each other in the event that a high-risk drinking situation occurs. If either one detects the return of old high-risk behaviors, both individuals immediately discuss with each other in a prearranged fashion the next step to take to prevent a relapse. This step differs, depending on the client and the situation. In some ways the simplest yet most drastic response is to notify the therapist. Frequently a brief phone conversation with the therapist suffices, but sometimes early in treatment or under unusual circumstances a session should be scheduled immediately.

In the dialogue that follows, the client has been sober for only 3 weeks. The couple had agreed to call the therapist if the precursors for relapse appeared, because both felt as if they needed the therapist's direct assistance during the early stages of recovery. The therapist was called by the wife, Maria, who stated that Phil had been withdrawing from her for several days. She made the decision to call when he refused to take his disulfiram for the second day in a row. Note that the therapist responds by scheduling a session as soon as possible, reinforcing the wife for following the Early Warning System plan, exploring the reasons for the appearance of the precursors or triggers now, reminding the client about his reinforcers for staying sober, and offering a clear plan for resolving the problem.

THERAPIST: I'm glad you both could come in tonight. Phil, when I talked to Maria this morning she seemed concerned about your refusal to take Antabuse the last couple of days.

CLIENT: I'm not drinking. I just don't want to take Antabuse.

THERAPIST: What's happening right now that makes you not want to take the Antabuse?

CLIENT: I feel like I can do it on my own. I don't need to take it.

THERAPIST: And why do you feel you don't need it?

CLIENT: I'm not drinking and I don't plan on drinking. So why should I take it?

THERAPIST: Uh-huh. Well, remember just over a month ago when we first started working together? You told me you would stay sober without taking the Antabuse for 7 days, but you only made it 5. So there have been times in the past when you haven't been able to attain your goal of abstinence. I hope this won't be the case now. But, we did make an agreement earlier to take the Antabuse for at least a minimum of 30 days. I'm curious. What is going on right now in your life to make you go back on your contract?

CLIENT: I'm not going back on it; I just don't need it.

WIFE: Well, let me tell you what's been going on. He's been moping around the house day and night, ignoring the kids, and snapping at me. Something is wrong.

THERAPIST: What's going on, Phil? Have you been a little upset lately; a little short-tempered? Often, 2 to 3 weeks after people stop drinking, their body chemistry is changing, and mood swings occur more frequently. Some of this is anticipated, like we talked about earlier. But this seems to be a little more radical or intense than normal. Also, as both of you well know, moping around and snapping at everybody have been some of your precursors to drinking in the past. Maria, it sounded on the phone like you recognized these as possible antecedents, but, just as we'd planned, you waited until 2 days of Antabuse were missed in a row before calling.

WIFE: I was glad we set that up. I wouldn't have known exactly what to do otherwise.

THERAPIST: You did a fine job, Maria.

Note: The therapist takes the opportunity to reinforce the wife for following the Early Warning System plan. The therapist knows that it is crucial to continue exploring *why* the client stopped taking his Antabuse.

THERAPIST: Phil, is there something going on that we need to know about?

CLIENT: I don't know. Why don't you ask her? She seems to be the authority on everything.

THERAPIST: Well, I really would rather ask you. You're the one that made the decision to quit drinking, and now you're the one who's made the decision to stop taking the Antabuse. I think it is fine to stop taking Antabuse at a certain point. I'm just not sure that this is the best time to do it without any discussion.

CLIENT: To be honest with you . . . I'm tired of not being able to "do anything right." I thought things were going to get better. Maria keeps bringing up my past drinking and some of the things I did. She doesn't trust me.

WIFE: I trust you more than I used to.

CLIENT: I thought that if I stopped drinking, and I started taking this Antabuse, things were going to get better. I was going to be happier. We both were.

THERAPIST: Well, how long have you been sober, Phil?

CLIENT: Almost 3 weeks.

THERAPIST: OK. And how many years did you drink?

CLIENT: Five years, maybe six. I don't know.

THERAPIST: That's a long history of drinking. It's going to take a while for the rest of your life to catch up with your quitting. So try not to get too discouraged. I know that one of the reasons why you wanted to quit was so you could be back home with Maria and the kids. I imagine your life now must be happier than when you were staying in that hotel room, isn't it?

CLIENT: Yeah.

Note: The therapist encourages the client to stay optimistic, and reminds him about his reinforcers for staying sober.

THERAPIST: So, where do you want to go from here?

CLIENT: Well, I definitely don't want to mess everything up. Maybe I'm just mad.

THERAPIST: It's okay to be mad. But let's learn how to handle the anger more effectively. It sounds like the two of you are definitely ready for your next session on marital communication skills training. We can do that before you leave today. You both need to find ways to comfortably express your feelings toward each other, even if they are difficult things to say. And Maria, it sounds like we may need to practice again being very supportive and reinforcing if Phil goes back on his Antabuse. Reminding him about his past problems is definitely not going to help right now. And Phil, if you'd like, I could review all the advantages of taking Antabuse.

Note: The therapist reminds the disulfiram monitor of the importance of being extremely supportive, and makes plans to conduct a much-needed communication skills training session before they leave. Finally, he offers to review the benefits to being on disulfiram.

CLIENT: No, I don't need to go over that again. OK. I'll take it the rest of the 30 days. But no promises after that.

THERAPIST: That's fine. Let's take it one step at a time. We will reevaluate the Antabuse at the end of your 30 days. Now let's figure out a healthy way for the two of you to express your anger toward each other.

The important issue in this dialogue is that the wife responded according to the Early Warning System plan, and phoned the therapist once the husband refused his disulfiram for the second straight day. In turn, the therapist promptly scheduled a session, and explored with the client the reasons why he was breaking his contract. This timely intervention may have prevented a relapse. Although the immediate crisis was over, the therapist knew that it was critical to teach the couple a new way to communicate with each other when they were angry.

It is very common to see a test at some point during the early part of therapy. It can appear in many forms, and it is not necessarily initiated by the client. As mentioned earlier, it does not have to revolve around a disulfiram issue. Renewed contact with one's drinking triggers can be the behavior designated to set the Early Warning System plan into motion.

Cognitive Restructuring to Prevent Relapse

In the previous dialogue, the couple was trained to respond to early warning signs or triggers by calling their therapist. As noted, the client was early in the recovery process, and such a step was deemed necessary for them. Eventually clients reach a stage in recovery where they do not need to call their therapist every time they have thoughts or urges to drink. Instead they rely on a cognitive behavioral technique called cognitive restructuring that already was introduced in the drink-refusal training section of Chapter 6.

To review, cognitive restructuring is a procedure used to identify and change maladaptive thought patterns. Common examples of the negative thoughts of individuals experiencing urges to drink are:

- "It's too difficult to face it anymore without a drink."
- "I'm sure I can stop after just one or two."
- "I can't help it. I'm an alcoholic."
- "I've already blown it. I might as well keep drinking."
- "I've been doing so well. I deserve a drink."

Turn to the internal triggers section of the client's initial functional analysis (see Appendix 2.A) to demonstrate readily the negative thought patterns that have led to drinking in the past. Once clients are made aware of this connection, they typically can generate additional negative beliefs unique to their own situation. The next task is to teach them adaptive ways to respond to these relapse triggers. Cognitive restructuring is geared specifically first to provide a *thought* that competes with the maladaptive, drinking-prone one. This positive thought should, in turn, elicit positive feelings. So in the future when clients find themselves repeating their typical negative statements that routinely result in alcohol consumption, ideally they will automatically substitute a positive, healthy alternative statement that promotes self confidence. Examples include:

- "Do I really want to spoil it? I've been doing so well. I know I'll feel better about myself if I don't drink."
- "I don't really need that drink. That's my old way of thinking. I actually have a lot of things to feel good about now!"

As mentioned in Chapter 6, sometimes it is helpful to follow the positive thought with an alternative *behavior*. This behavior could be a walk, a phone call to a friend, an AA meeting, a nap, or a wide variety of other nondrinking activities. Relapse prevention appears to be most successful when the behavior is preplanned, and when it supplies most of the short-term positive consequences that historically were associated with the client's drinking.

◆ ◆

In summary, this chapter has presented several options for relapse prevention training: the CRA Functional Analysis (Relapse Version), an examination of the behavioral chain leading to relapse, implementation of an Early Warning System, and cognitive restructuring of thoughts that lead to drinking. The choice of which technique to use, or how many, depends primarily on your preference and the client's unique situation. Regardless, the important message is that relapse prevention work really begins early in the treatment process, since each technique is built upon an awareness of one's drinking triggers.

APPENDIXES 10.A–10.B

Appendix 10.A   CRA FUNCTIONAL ANALYSIS FOR DRINKING BEHAVIOR (RELAPSE VERSION)

Triggers		Behavior	Short-Term Positive Consequences	Long-Term Negative Consequences
External	**Internal**			
1. Who were you with when you drank?	1. What were you thinking about right before you drank?	1. What were you drinking?	1. What did you like about drinking with _____? (who)	1. What were the negative results of your drinking in each of these areas: a) Interpersonal:
2. Where were you when you drank?	2. What were you feeling physically right before you drank?	2. How much did you drink?	2. What did you like about drinking _____? (where)	b) Physical:
			3. What did you like about drinking _____? (when)	c) Emotional:

3. When did you drink?

3. What were you feeling emotionally right before you drank?

3. Over how long a period of time did you drink?

4. What were some of the pleasant thoughts you had while you were drinking?

5. What were some of the pleasant physical feelings you had while you were drinking?

6. What were some of the pleasant emotional feelings you had while you were drinking?

d) Legal:

e) Job:

f) Financial:

g) Other:

Appendix 10.B CRA FUNCTIONAL ANALYSIS FOR DRINKING BEHAVIOR (RELAPSE VERSION)

External ⟶ Triggers ⟶ Internal		Behavior	Short-Term Positive Consequences	Long-term Negative Consequences
1. Who were you with when you drank? *Max*	1. What were you thinking about right before you drank? *How unfair it was to be laid off. I deserved a good drunk.*	1. What were you drinking? *Beer*	1. What did you like about drinking with _Max_? (who) *We went on & on about being laid off. It felt good.*	1. What were the negative results of your drinking in each of these areas: a) Interpersonal: *Wife is angry at me.* *(parents are, too)*
2. Where were you when you drank? *Max's house*	2. What were you feeling physically right before you drank? *Sick - upset stomach, tense.*	2. How much did you drink? *2 1/2–3 cases*	2. What did you like about drinking _at Max's house_? (where) *Nobody bothers us there.*	b) Physical: *I feel sick.*
			3. What did you like about drinking _after being laid off_? (when) *It felt good to be putting down the company.*	c) Emotional: *I feel like a failure.*

194

3. Over how long a period of time did you drink?

5 days

3. When did you drink?

Friday—as soon as we got laid off.

3. What were you feeling emotionally right before you drank?

mad, hurt

4. What were some of the pleasant thoughts you had while you were drinking?

We were getting revenge.

5. What were some of the pleasant physical feelings you had while you were drinking?

Felt relaxed; no knot in stomach.

6. What were some of the pleasant emotional feelings you had while you were drinking?

Satisfaction, revenge.

d) Legal:

—

e) Job:

Wasn't out looking for a new job.

f) Financial:

Spent money on beer.

g) Other:

11

The Big Picture

C RA is more than a set of therapeutic interventions; it is a philosophy regarding the best way to assist individuals in making lasting behavior changes. But a fair number of beginning therapists almost become distracted by CRA's broad array of behavioral techniques. As a result, they sometimes lose sight of the big picture; namely, that the goal is always to move toward making a nondrinking lifestyle more rewarding than drinking. In training CRA therapists over the years to accomplish this objective, several relatively common "mistakes" have become apparent. A brief description of these difficulties and their solutions follows.

COMMON MISTAKES MADE
WHEN IMPLEMENTING CRA

Losing Sight of the Client's Reinforcers

The importance of always being aware of a client's reinforcers cannot be stressed enough. Dramatic changes in an individual's lifestyle will be short-lived if he or she is not reinforced in the process. Unfortunately, it is fairly easy to become narrowly focused on "fixing" a client's drinking problem, without stopping to check for the link with the person's reinforcers. A case in point was a therapist who assisted a client in obtaining an interview for an excellent job in a nearby city. The problem was that the relocation would limit the time that this divorced client would be able to spend with his two young children. The client had made it clear on his functional analysis that his visits with his children were one of his greatest reinforcers. The therapist had been so concerned about removing the client from his current high-risk drinking environment that he had neglected to explore the full extent of what the client would lose in the process. Usually one can avoid this oversight by reviewing the client's functional analysis or Goals of Counseling form periodically to recall the motivators. Another option is to simply ask on a regular basis, "What are the client's reinforcers?"

Some CRA therapists report even greater difficulty identifying a client's reinforcers in the first place. A student in training once insisted that it was impossible to find reinforcers to motivate certain clients. She described working in a women's prison with inmates who were mandated to attend alcohol treatment groups, but who stated they had no intention of curbing their drinking once released. By focusing on the clients' negative verbal behavior and losing sight of the big picture, this therapist was unable to see at least one primary reinforcer in these women's lives: staying out of prison. Based on their histories, it was clear that resuming old drinking habits was, in essence, paving the way for their return to prison.

Of course, once a therapist sees this connection between drinking and the loss of an important reinforcer, the message still must be conveyed to the client. You can always fall back on the "Columbo" routine: Act naive and use paradoxical questions. For instance, say, "I don't quite understand. I thought you said you hated prison and never wanted to return. By going back to your old drinking habits you almost guarantee another visit." Or you might try, "I guess you must really like me, because it seems that ultimately your goal is to come back and visit me." If it is clear that being home with one's family is a reinforcer, this potential loss could be made even more obvious. You could ask, "Didn't you say you wanted to go home and spend time with your husband and kids? If you fall back into your drinking and drugging routine you're headed for the same kind of trouble that landed you in jail in the first place. But the next time you'll probably end up being away from your family even longer."

The moral of the story is that the reinforcers for addressing a drinking problem are always there; it is simply a matter of sifting through the information provided by clients to find them. The next step is discovering a way to utilize your findings so that you are collaborating with clients to achieve their objectives.

Failing to Involve Concerned Others in Treatment

Another mistake made by therapists is neglecting to involve Concerned Others in the treatment process. There appear to be several reasons for this. Some therapists simply feel uncomfortable including the spouses of problem drinkers, for they believe they lack the necessary therapy skills for work with couples. This was addressed briefly in Chapter 9 (CRA Marital Therapy), and is described fully in Meyers, Dominguez, & Smith (in press).

Due to the sizeable menu of available CRA procedures, some therapists believe that they have a sufficient number of tools to treat a client without including another player. In some ways this is analogous to losing sight of a client's reinforcers, for a Concerned Other often controls access to many of these. Depending on the relationship of the Concerned Other to the client, these reinforcers may include emotional support, children, a sexual relationship, recreational opportunities, and companionship. Given this, and the fact that this individual typically is extremely interested in seeing the client's drinking problem improve, the Concerned Other can be a powerful addition to the treatment program.

More often than not there appears to be a substantial payoff for making the extra effort to involve a Concerned Other in the therapy. Early research demonstrated that those clients who had a Concerned Other participate in their treatment had better outcomes than those who did not (Azrin et al., 1982). In part, the effect may have been due to the Concerned Other receiving communication training. Perhaps an even greater component, however, was the inclusion of the Concerned Other in the partner's change process. It enabled the Concerned Other to be aware of the therapeutic strategies and goals as they evolved, and to participate in some of the decision making.

By way of an example, examine the case of an alcohol-dependent woman in treatment who decided to work on her goals of improving her relationship with her sister and enhancing her self-esteem. She efficiently arranged to address both goals simultaneously by joining her sister in her after-dinner walks three nights a week. Initially her husband had not been involved in her treatment program. He became very upset regarding what he perceived to be his wife's loss of interest in him, and her preference for doing anything in the evening except spend time with him. Without an understanding of her treatment plan it was impossible for him to recognize the significant role this activity played in rearranging her drinking lifestyle. Once included in the therapy process he was able to fully support his wife's walks with her sister, and to generate additional suggestions for goal-directed strategies.

Neglecting to Emphasize the Importance of Having a Satisfying Social Life

At times therapists minimize the importance of helping clients establish a satisfying social life, for they assume that individuals are skilled at having fun. But as noted in Chapter 8 (Social and Recreational Counseling), many clients are ill prepared to find new activities and friends that do not involve alcohol. As a result they elect to ignore that part of their lives initially. But social and recreational activities are significant reinforcers for most people. Consequently, clients who are not trained to develop nondrinking social activities eventually react in one of two ways. Some continue to exclude these activities from their lives, and as a result become bored or depressed. This was the case with John, a client who maintained sobriety for several months, but who totally withdrew socially. He repeatedly told his therapist that he was staying away from trouble. He refused to work on establishing a new social network, insisting that the office was enough of a social life for him. Not surprisingly, over the months he became more and more despondent. He started showing many physical signs of depression as well, including appetite loss and sleep disturbance. John insisted that he was fine, but one day his wife called to report that he had not been home for 48 hours. He was drunk and seeking refuge in a motel room downtown.

Some clients attempt to resume their previous drinking-related social activities and friendships, but without imbibing themselves. All too often it is not long before the powerful social cues prevail, and the good-intentioned client is drinking again. So making a point of showing a client how to develop new recreational activities and find supportive friends is a critical part of the CRA package.

Not Stressing the Necessity of Having a Meaningful Job

Another way in which a client's "community" is not rearranged to support a nondrinking lifestyle is by focusing exclusively on a client's drinking status, while ignoring the fact that the person does not have meaningful employment. During a supervision session years ago, a new CRA therapist proudly reported that his client was doing extremely well. He had been sober for 3 weeks, and had faithfully attended every session. When the therapist was asked how this unemployed client's job search was proceeding, the young therapist froze and muttered, "Oh, right. A job. We haven't quite gotten around to working on that yet." It was clear that the therapist had not been considering the big picture, for the probability of the client returning to alcohol once his meager funds ran out was extremely high. Without a mechanism in place for financially ensuring continued access to valuable reinforcers, the success story would be short-lived.

The situation can be equally problematic if a client possesses a job but is unhappy with it. Assuming the individual remains in the position, he or she is at risk for becoming depressed and withdrawing, or for finding maladaptive ways to reward him- or herself for having to deal with the stress or drudgery of work. This paves the way for resorting to drinking again.

Inadequately Monitoring the Client's Contact with Triggers

It is easy to underestimate both the strength of a client's drinking triggers and their frequency of occurrence in the environment. As mentioned earlier, they can be present in specific social environments, or in certain types of jobs held previously by a client. With regard to the latter, let us turn to a therapist who reported that her client was going on his first real job interview. Upon inquiring, we soon discovered that the position was for a plumber, the same line of work that the client had been in for years. And although the client had impressive credentials for the position and felt self-assured about obtaining it, it was clear from his functional analysis that a plumbing job would place him directly back into contact with many of his drinking triggers. Furthermore, the client later admitted that he did not enjoy that type of work anymore, and he only pursued it because of the high salary. With all things considered, a plumbing job seemed to be the perfect setup for a relapse.

Certainly it is not possible nor even desirable to protect a client from ever facing a drinking trigger. The recommended strategy is to regularly assist a client in rearranging his or her environment so that contact with triggers is minimized, and to problem-solve mechanisms for coping with those that cannot be avoided.

Not Checking for Generalizability of Skills

One of the well-recognized limitations of behavioral skills training is the problem of generalizability to the client's real world. Many individuals are quite proficient at performing, for example, newly learned drink-refusal and problem-solving skills during therapy sessions. Unfortunately they have great difficulty incorporating these skills into their everyday lives. Consequently, you should not assume that clients are applying these new procedures, and if they are, that they are applying them correctly. So have them track and report the specific times and places in which they attempted to apply the procedures during the week, and discuss any unforeseen difficulties they experienced. Ask them to reenact several of the real-world events during the session, so that their skill level can be observed at a time somewhat removed from the actual training.

In some cases clients do not give themselves the opportunity to put newly learned skills into practice, because they actively avoid the situations that are likely to require them. Lance was a perfect example of this, for he stayed away from all people and places even remotely associated with alcohol. This made him extremely vulnerable on an occasion in which he accidently found himself in a drinking environment. He had great difficulty refusing a drink, because he had not built up his confidence and skill with a series of past successes. Consequently, it is advisable to have clients gradually place themselves in progressively more challenging situations, in order to develop their skills and enhance their self-esteem.

Being Reluctant to Suggest the Use of Disulfiram

For a variety of reasons, therapists have been known to avoid the suggestion of disulfiram as an adjunct to treatment. Some are reluctant to make the recommendation because it "complicates" therapy; namely, a physician and possibly laboratory tests need to be involved. Others are opposed to what they perceive as a client relying on a medication to stop drinking. Typically these therapists are unaware of the fact that disulfiram is only a short-term supplement to treatment that generally is restricted to the 90-day high-risk period. Furthermore, during that same time many strategies are also being taught to modify drinking behaviors.

Some therapists offer the rationale that clients will view disulfiram as too harsh a measure. With probing it becomes apparent that these therapists have met with resistance to the idea from some clients in the past. Although it is clearly the case that disulfiram is not appropriate for every alcohol abuser, client resistance alone should not dissuade you from recommending it when indicated. Those clients who are resistant typically fear the negative consequences of disulfiram. Many have heard horror stories from experienced friends. But as noted in Chapter 4 (Disulfiram Use Within

CRA) the negative consequences will only materialize if clients drink while taking disulfiram. By reminding them of this critical element one often can appeal to their level of commitment and enhance their motivation in the process.

CRA: SOMETHING FOR EVERYBODY

CRA therapists sometimes are reluctant to inform other counselors about CRA simply because they do not have a behavioral or cognitive-behavioral orientation. In actuality there are variations of several CRA procedures that already are utilized by more traditional substance abuse counselors. For example, both CRA and 12-step counselors rely upon types of modeling and chaining. Positive reinforcement, one of the cornerstones of CRA, is utilized by 12-step therapists in the form of a 30-day chip.

Furthermore, there are CRA procedures that readily could be added to a traditional counselor's methods. Assume, for instance, that a therapist believes AA is an essential treatment ingredient. The client may even believe this as well, but the potential benefits of AA will never be realized if the client does not actually attend meetings. The CRA procedures that can help a therapist achieve this objective include Systematic Encouragement, Reinforcer Access, and Reinforcer Sampling (see Chapter 8: Social and Recreational Counseling). These empirically tested, successful procedures rely upon a supportive and nonconfrontational approach that encourages a client to try new activities.

Another example of a CRA procedure that has broad applicability is Sobriety Sampling. Some therapists initially are resistant to the notion of a client contracting for time-limited sobriety, for they believe that motivated individuals should be prepared from the start to commit to a lifetime of abstinence. But often clients are more willing to attempt shorter periods of sobriety. Interestingly, frequently these grow into a chain of shorter periods, such that a day evolves into weeks, months, or even years of abstinence (Miller & Page, 1991). So Sobriety Sampling aptly fits the model that an individual can only stay sober one day at a time.

If other therapists are not convinced about CRA's potential contribution to their own approach at this point, do the only logical thing: Appeal to their reinforcers! Typically most therapists will say that they are working in the field because they "want to help people." If helping clients stay sober and live productively is paramount, then present the treatment outcome literature that shows CRA's outstanding record for accomplishing this goal (Miller et al., 1995).

As noted in Chapter 1: History of the Community Reinforcement Approach, for the most part CRA has been used with alcohol-abusive and alcohol-dependent populations. More recently it has proven successful in the treatment of cocaine dependence (Higgins et al., 1991, 1993), and research trials in progress are testing its efficacy with heroin addicts and homeless individuals. The flexibility of the approach readily lends itself to a variety of problems that are only now being explored.

References

Azrin, N.H. (1976). Improvements in the community reinforcement approach to alcoholism. *Behaviour Research and Therapy*, 14, 339-348.

Azrin, N.H., & Besalel, V.A. (1980). *Job club counselor's manual*. Baltimore, MD: University Press.

Azrin, N.H., Naster, B.J., & Jones, R. (1973). Reciprocity counseling: A rapid learning-based procedure for marital counseling. *Behaviour Research and Therapy*, 11, 365-382.

Azrin, N.H., Sisson, W., Meyers, R., & Godley, M. (1982). Alcoholism treatment by disulfiram and community reinforcement therapy. *Journal of Behavior Therapy and Experimental Psychiatry*, 13, 105-112.

Brownell, K.D., Marlatt, G.A., Lichtenstein, E., & Wilson, G.T. (1986). Understanding and preventing relapse. *American Psychologist*, 41, 765-782.

Budney, A.J., Higgins, S.T., Delaney, D.D., Kent, L., & Bickel, W.K. (1991). Contingent reinforcement of abstinence with individuals abusing cocaine and marijuana. *Journal of Applied Behavior Analysis*, 24, 657-665.

Cahalan, D., Cisin, I.H., & Crossley, H.M. (1969). *American drinking practices: A national study of drinking behavior and attitudes* (Rutgers Center on Alcohol Studies, Monograph No. 6).

Childress, A.R., Hole, A.V., Ehrman, R.N., Robbins, S.J., McLellan, A.T., & O'Brien, C.P. (1993). Cue reactivity and cue reactivity interventions in drug dependence. *National Institute on Drug Abuse Research Monograph Series*, 137, 73-95.

D'Zurilla, T., & Goldfried, M. (1971). Problem solving and behavior modification. *Journal of Abnormal Psychology*, 78, 107-126.

Federal Register (1989). Rules and regulations, 21 CFR Part 291, Food and Drug Administration, Vol. 54, No. 40. Rockville, MD. National Institute on Drug Abuse.

Hawkins, J.D., Catalano, R.F., Gillmore, M.R., & Wells, E.A. (1989). Skills training for drug abusers: Generalization, maintenance, and effects on drug use. *Journal of Consulting and Clinical Psychology*, 57, 559-563.

Higgins, S.T., Budney, A.J., Bickel, W.K., Hughes, J.R., Foerg, F., & Badger, G. (1993). Achieving cocaine abstinence with a behavioral approach. *American Journal of Psychiatry*, 150(5), 763-769.

Higgins, S.T., Delaney, D.D., Budney, A.J., Bickel, W.K., Hughes, J.R., & Foerg, F. (1991). A behavioral approach to achieving initial cocaine abstinence. *American Journal of Psychiatry*, 148, 1218-1224.

Hunt, G.M., & Azrin, N.H. (1973). A community-reinforcement approach to alcoholism. *Behaviour Research and Therapy*, 11, 91-104.

Jellinek, E.M. (1960). The disease concept of alcoholism. New Haven: College and University Press.

Jellinek, R.A. (1952). Phases of alcohol addiction. *Quarterly Journal of Studies on Alcohol*, 13, 673-684.

Mallams, J.H., Godley, M.D., Hall, G.M., & Meyers, R.J. (1982). A social-systems approach to resocializing alcoholics in the community. *Journal of Studies on Alcohol*, 43, 1115-1123.

Marlatt, G.A. (1980). Relapse prevention: A self-control program for the treatment of addictive behaviors. Unpublished manuscript.

Marlatt, G.A., & Gordon, J.R. (Eds.). (1985). *Relapse prevention: Maintenance strategies in the treatment of addictive behaviors.* New York: Guilford Press.

Martin, J.C. Father. (1972). *Chalk talk* [Film]. Available from FMS Productions, Carpenteria, CA.

McLellan, A.T., Luborsky, L., Woody, G.E., & O'Brien, C.P. (1980). An improved diagnostic evaluation instrument for substance abuse patients: The Addiction Severity Index. *Journal of Nervous and Mental Disease*, 168, 26-33.

Meyers, R.J., Dominguez, T., & Smith, J.E. (in press). Community reinforcement training with concerned others. In V.B. Hasselt & M. Hersen (Eds.), *Source of psychological treatment manuals for adults.* New York: Plenum Press.

Miller, W.R. (1993). The Stages of Change Readiness and Treatment Eagerness Scale, Version 6. Unpublished research instruments. University of New Mexico.

Miller, W.R., Brown, J.M., Simpson, T.L., Handmaker, N.S., Bien, T.H., Luckie, L.F., Montgomery, H.A., Hester, R.K., & Tonigan, J.S. (1995). What works? A methodological analysis of the alcohol treatment outcome literature. In R.K. Hester & W.R. Miller (Eds.), *Handbook of alcoholism treatment approaches: Effective alternatives* (2nd ed.). Needham, MA: Allyn & Bacon.

Miller, W.R., & Marlatt, G.A. (1984). *Manual for the Comprehensive Drinker Profile.* Odessa, FL: Psychological Assessment Resources.

Miller, W.R., & Marlatt, G.A. (1987). *Comprehensive Drinker Profile— Manual supplement.* Odessa, FL: Psychological Assessment Resources.

Miller, W.R., & Page, A.C. (1991). Warm turkey: Other routes to abstinence. *Journal of Substance Abuse Treatment, 8,* 227-232.

Miller, W.R., Tonigan, J.S., & Longabaugh, R. (1994). DrInC: An instrument for assessing adverse consequences of alcohol abuse. Unpublished manuscript. University of New Mexico.

Miller, W.R., Westerberg, V.S., & Waldron, H.B. (1995). Evaluating alcohol problems in adults and adolescents. In R.K. Hester & W.R. Miller (Eds.), *Handbook of alcoholism treatment approaches: Effective alternatives* (2nd ed.). Needham, MA: Allyn & Bacon.

Monti, P., Abrams, D., Kadden, R., & Cooney, N. (1989). *Treating alcohol dependence: A coping skills training guide.* New York: Guilford Press.

Prochaska, J.O., & DiClemente, C.C. (1986). Toward a comprehensive model of change. In W.R. Miller & N. Heather (Eds.), *Treating addictive behaviors: Processes of change* (pp. 3-27). New York: Plenum Press.

Sisson, R.W., & Azrin, N.H. (1986). Family-member involvement to initiate and promote treatment of problem drinkers. *Behavior Therapy and Experimental Psychiatry, 17,* 15-21.

Sisson, R.W., & Mallams, J.H. (1981). The use of systematic encouragement and community access procedures to increase attendance at Alcoholics Anonymous and Al-Anon meetings. *American Journal of Drug and Alcohol Abuse, 8*(3), 371-376.

Stuart, R.B. (1969). Operant-interpersonal treatment for marital discord. *Journal of Consulting and Clinical Psychology, 33,* 675-682.

Index

A

Abbott, P., 13
Abrams, D., 115
Alcoholics Anonymous (AA)
    clinical studies contrasting CRA,
        and, 1–6, 8–14
    incorporation of CRA procedures,
        202
Antabuse. *See* Disulfiram
Antecedents. *See also* Assessment,
        Behavioral skills training,
        Social and recreational
        counseling
    drinking behavior
        disulfiram use, and, 63
        early warning system, 186–189
        external triggers, 21–25, 113–117,
            129–131
        high-risk situations, 113–117,
            129–131
        identification of, 21–25
        internal triggers, 21–25, 117–119
        need to adequately monitor, 200
        relapse, and, 181–184
        sobriety sampling, and, 46–49,
            54
    nondrinking behavior, 29–31
Assessment
    background and substance use
        information, 19–20
    functional analysis
        description and objectives, 20–
        21

drinking behavior, 25–26
    negative consequences, 27–29
    short-term positive conse-
        quences, 26–27, 181–184
forms
    drinking behavior (initial
        assessment), 34–37, 113, 117
    nondrinking behavior, 38–41
    standardized instruments, 19
identifying antecedents to drink-
    ing, 21–25
intakes, 19–20
motivation, identification, and
    enhancement, 17–19
nondrinking
    negative consequences, 31–32
    positive consequences, 32–33
    positive triggers for, 29–31
Avoidance of high-risk drinking
    situations, 129–131
Azrin, N.H., 1–6, 10, 11, 20, 122, 148,
    198

B

Besalel, V.A., 122
Behavioral skills training. *See also*
        Marital therapy
    application to everyday life, 200–
        201
    communication skills training,
        102–105
    drink-refusal training

Behavioral skills training (*cont'd*)
  enlisting social support, 111–113
  clinical study, use in, 4–5
  refusing drinks assertively, 115–117
  restructuring negative thoughts, 117–119, 189–190
  reviewing high-risk situations, 113–115
  problem-solving training
  problem-solving steps, 106–111
  simulated blackboard presentation, 120
  role plays, 75, 105, 112, 114,124–125, 141, 144–145
Bickel, W.K., 7, 8
Budney, A.J., 7, 8

C

Cocaine dependency, use of CRA, 7–10
Communication skills training. *See* Behavioral skills training
Concerned Other. *See also* Marital therapy
  clinical studies, involvement in, 4–7, 11
  disulfiram use, and, 11–13, 63, 67–70, 72–77, 131–134
  failure to involve, 198–199
  involvement in nondrinking social activities, 140, 145
  motivation for treatment, and, 6–7, 18–20, 131–134
  reinforcers, 19
  relapse prevention, and, 186–189
  substance abuse by, 19–20
Consequences. *See also* Assessment
  of drinking, 26–29
  of nondrinking, 31–33
Contingency management, use of CRA with, 7–10
Cooney, N., 115
CRA (Community Reinforcement Approach). *See also* Assessment, Disulfiram, Job

counseling, Marital therapy, Relapse prevention, Sobriety sampling, Social and recreational counseling, Treatment plan
  basic components, 1, 17
  broad applicability, 202–203
  early trials, inpatients, 1–3
  early trials, outpatients, 3–5
  early warning monitoring system, 136
  environmental contingencies, role of, 1
  goals, 196
  group treatment, 3, 14
  homeless population, 14–15
  implementation, common mistakes
    failure to involve Concerned Others, 198–199
    failure to stress need for meaningful job, 199–200
    inadequate monitoring of client's triggers, 200
    losing sight of reinforcers, 196–198
    neglecting importance of social life, 199
    not checking for generalizability of skills, 200–201
    reluctance to suggest use of disulfiram, 201–202
  marital status, effect of, 5
  ongoing studies, 10–15
  philosophy, 1
  relaxation training, 4, 7
  social club, 2, 5–6, 145–146
  social systems approach, 1
  therapy time, 2–4, 7–9, 13, 14
  vs. Standard Treatment (AA), 1–6, 8–14

D

Delaney, D.D., 7, 8
Disulfiram (Antabuse)
  ability to take, 11–12, 14–15

administration procedure, 3–5, 74–77
advantages, 59, 62–64
characteristics, 57, 59
client consent form, 64, 78
client contract, 64–67, 71–72
clinical studies, use in, 3–5, 9, 11–12, 14–15
concerned other, involvement of, 4, 11–13, 63, 67–70, 72–77, 131–134
effective treatment component, 59–62
family physician, involvement of, 64
obtaining client commitment, 58–62, 64–67
monitoring system, 3–5, 72–77
recognizing need for, 57–59
refusal of, 64–67
sample letter to physician, 79
therapist, reluctance to suggest use, 201–202
willingness of client to take, 11–12, 14–15
Drink refusal training. *See* Behavioral skills training
Drug abuse, use of CRA, 7–10, 13, 203
Duration training, 129–131
D'Zurilla, T., 106

F

Family member. *See also* Concerned Other
initiation of treatment by, 6–7
Functional Analysis. *See* Assessment, Relapse prevention

G

Godley, M., 3, 5, 10, 11
Goldfried, M., 106

H

Hall, G.M., 5
Happiness Scale. *See* Treatment plan
Heroin abuse, use of CRA, 13
Higgins, S.T., 7, 8
Hunt, G.M., 1, 20

I

Independence training, 135–137
Intake information, 19–20

J

Job Club Counselor's Manual, 122–123, 125
Job counseling
avoiding jobs with high relapse potential, 123
completing job applications, 123–124
developing a résumé, 122–123
general description, 122
generating job leads, 124
interview rehearsal, 125
learning how to keep a job, 125–126
purpose, 121–122
telephone skills training, 124–125

K

Kadden, R., 115
Kent, L., 7, 8

M

Mallams, J.H., 5,138
Marijuana use, 7–10
Marital status, effect on treatment, 4–5
Marital therapy
ambivalence toward change, 162–163
applicability, 148
communication skills
art of negotiation, 167–170

Marital therapy (*cont'd*)
  basics, 163–164
  ending the session, 170
  new skills, 165–166
  practicing requests, 164–165
  role of the listener, 166–167
  using Perfect Marriage Form,
    164–165
  Daily Reminder to Be Nice form,
    158–160, 179
  Marriage Happiness Scale, 149–
    153, 171–173
  need for, 147–148
  Perfect Marriage form, description
    and purpose, 153
  forms, 174–178
  practicing requests with, 164–165
  session goals, 160–162
  setting positive expectations, 148–
    149
Marlatt, G.A., 19,44,62
Meyers, R.J., 3, 5, 10, 11, 13, 14
Miller, W.R., 10, 16, 19
Monti, P., 102,115
Motivation. *See also* Antecedents to
    drinking, Assessment,
    Reinforcers
  enhancement, 17–18
  concerned other, involvement and,
    6–7, 18–20, 131–134
  questionnaires, 19
  setting positive expectations, 18
Motivation reversal, 129, 131–135
Multiple-drug dependence, 8–10

O

Operant reinforcement theory, 2

P

Paradoxical intention. *See* Motiva-
    tion reversal
Problem-solving training. *See*
    Behavioral skills training
Prompt rule, use with nonresponsive
    client, 128–129

R

Reinforcers. *See also* Assessment
  access, 143
  financial, 9–10
  functional analysis, and,
    20–21
  identification, 18, 197
  intangible, 118
  material, 7–8, 14
  motivation, and, 17–19
  motivation reversal, and, 135
  need for constant awareness of,
    196–198
  positive reinforcer, definition, 17–18
  sampling, 140–141
Relapse prevention
  behavioral chain leading to
    relapse, 185–186
  cognitive restructuring, 189–190
  CRA Functional Analysis for
    Drinking Behavior (Relapse
    Version) form, 180–184, 192–
    195
  early warning system, 186–189,
    135–137
  heroin treatment, 13

S

Significant Other. *See* Concerned
    Other
Sisson, R.W., 3, 6, 10, 11
Smith, J.E., 14
Sobriety Sampling. *See also*
    Disulfiram
  advantages, 43
  applicability, 202
  client commitment, 43–46, 50–53,
    64–67
  confrontation, avoidance, 53–56
  introduction to client, 43–46
  purposes, 42–43
  resistant client, and, 50–53
  strategies for accomplishing goal,
    46–50, 53–55
  time-limited sobriety, 46–50

vs. abstinence as goal, 42, 55
Social and recreational counseling
concerned others, involvement in, 140
identifying alternate activities, 139–140
reinforcer access, 143
reinforcer sampling, 140–141
response priming, 143–145
social club, 2, 5–6, 145–146
social life and drinking, 138–139
systematic encouragement, 141–143
Solution orientation vs. problem orientation, 126–128
Standard treatment. *See* Alcoholics Anonymous
Stuart, R., 148
Systematic encouragement, 6

T

Treatment plan
Goals of Counseling form

basic rules for completing form, 84–86
description and purpose, 84
determine appropriate intervention, 86–89
planning for skills training, 89–92
potential problems completing form, 93–94
simplifying a complicated goal, 92–93
specifying an intervention, 86–89
Happiness Scale
explaining scale to client, 81–83
forms, 95–96
using scale throughout treatment, 83–84
review periodically, 119
Triggers. *See* Antecedents to drinking

W

Waldron, H.B., 16, 19
Westerberg, V.S., 16, 19